I dedicate this book to my parents who first set me on my life journey in the martial arts. I cannot thank them enough for their love, kindness, care, and support of me as I progressed onwards and upward from my first beginners class in Pak Mei Kung Fu.

They were always there to encourage me when I was discouraged, and to help me in the best way they could. They selflessly went without, so I never needed to. I love you both endlessly and cannot thank you enough.

Isometric Power Exercises for Martial Arts™

Build Superior Strength, Muscle and Martial Arts 'Firepower' Using the Proven System Bruce Lee Used

Published by

MajorVision International

2019

Approved by The World Isometric Exercise Association
www.TWiEA.com

▲ | TWiEA
The World Isometric Exercise Association

Copyright and Trademark Notice
© 2019 Brian Sterling-Vete and Helen Renée Wuorio All Rights Reserved

All material in this book is the property of, copyrighted, and trademarked to Brian Sterling-Vete and Helen Renée Wuorio, and/or MajorVision Ltd unless otherwise stated, AE&OE. Copyright and other intellectual property laws protect these materials. Reproduction, distribution, or transmission of the materials, in whole or in part, in any manner, without the prior written consent of the copyright holder is prohibited and is a violation of national and international copyright law.

The following names, exercises, and workout systems are the property of, copyright, and trademarked to Brian Sterling-Vete and Helen Renée, and/or MajorVision Ltd. ISOfitness™, The 70 Second Difference™, Adaptive Response™, Zero Footprint Workout™, ZFW™, Fitness on the Move™, FOM™, The ISO90™ Course, ISO90™, The SSASS Workout™, SSASS™, Dynamic Flexation™, The Bullworker Bible™, The Bullworker 90™, The Bullworker Compendium™, Workout at Work™, Doorway to Strength™, The TRISO90™ Course, TRISOmetrics™, The ISOmetric Bible™, Brian Sterling-Vete's Mental Martial Arts™, Tuxedo Warriors™, The Tuxedo Warrior™, The Pike, The Beast of Kane, Being American Married to a Brit, Paranormal Investigation - The Black Book of Scientific Ghost Hunting and How to Investigate Paranormal Phenomena, The Haunting of Lilford Hall™, Isometric Exercises for Nordic Walking and Trekking™ Pt.1, Isometric Exercises for Nordic Walking and Trekking™ Pt. 2, Isometric Power Exercises for Martial Arts™.

Artwork, designed by MAJORVISION.COM

Contents

Important General Safety and Health Guidelines

Introductions, Precautions and Thanks
- Precautions
- Thanks

1. **Isometrics, the Martial Arts and Bruce Lee**
2. **Exercise Science Overview**
    - Walking Vs Running as a Fat Burner
    - Walking, General Activity and N.E.A.T. - Non-Exercise Activity Thermogenesis
    - The Basic Types of Resistance Exercise
    - Isometrics
    - Isometric Exercise Science
    - The Standard Isometric Contraction
    - Workout Intensity
    - Technically, How Does Muscle Grow?
    - Rest and Recovery
    - Rest Time Between Exercises
    - Dynamic Flexation™
    - Isometric Exercises and Blood Pressure
3. **Improvised and Proprietary Isometric Exercise Equipment**
    - Securing the Iso-Bow® With Your Feet
4. **Direct Comparisons**
5. **Things to Remember Before You Begin**
    - Equipment
6. **About the Exercise Models**
7. **Exercise Resources**
8. **Conclusion**

Important General Safety and Health Guidelines

This section entitled, "Important General Safety and Health Guidelines," pertains to The ISOfitness™ Exercise System, and all books and publications about it not limited to but including The ISO90™ Course, Fitness on the Move™, The 70 Second Difference™, The Bullworker Bible™, The Sixty Second Ass Workout™, The Bullworker 90™ Course, The Bullworker Compendium™, Workout at Work™, The Doorway to Strength™, TRISOmetrics™, The TRISO90™ Course, the TRISOmetric™ system, The ISOmetric Bible™, Isometric Power Exercises for Martial Arts™, Isometric Exercises for Nordic Walking and Trekking™ Part 1., and Part 2., general and specific recommendations, suggestions, coaching, and advice, either written, verbal, in audio format, on video, written, or given, implied, or suggested the authors, from Brian Sterling-Vete, Helen Renée Wuorio, and the works thereof.

You should never begin any kind of sport, exercise system, workout plan, or diet modification, including everything contained in this book and any books mentioned in the beginning paragraph above unless you have consulted with and have the full approval of your medical doctor. Only your physician can accurately assess your current health status, and your ability to perform the exercises in the book and/or course. This is particularly important if you have any known or unknown pre-existing health issues, are pregnant, or believe that you may have other serious health conditions.

You must always have absolute approval from your physician/GP before starting. Please show all the material in the above courses, books, video/audio, online material, and their content to your physician and get their approval before you start.

All exercises, suggestions, recommendations, instructions, exercise plans, and dietary recommendations, either given or implied, are intended only as a reference, and they are no substitute for a qualified professional personal coach who can help you to plan an exercise and diet program appropriate for your age and physical condition. Never overexert yourself when performing any exercise. Stop exercising immediately and always consult your doctor and/or call the EMS immediately if you ever experience any pain, irregular heartbeat, shortness of breath, tightness in your chest/arms/fingers, faintness, nausea, or feelings of dizziness.

The exercises, courses, plans, and dietary recommendations in this book together with all those mentioned in all the books, general publications, online material, and videos mentioned in the names in paragraph 1 of this section, are not intended for use by children. Keep all exercise equipment out of the reach of children.

Always inspect any exercise equipment, and/or any/all other improvised or specifically made exercise equipment/materials, doors, door jambs, door frames, and anything else you use before each use to ensure its proper operation and to ensure that it is undamaged and safe. Do not use it unless all parts are free from wear, and it is functioning properly. Care should always be taken to avoid serious injury using any/all exercise equipment, and in all items, people, books, and courses mentioned in paragraph 1 of this section. Care should always be taken when getting into all exercise positions, on and off the floor, on and off chairs, on and off benches, on and off any other surface that might be used for exercise, including pieces of furniture, and in the use of all exercised equipment, either purpose-made or improvised.

The creators, writers, instructors, originators, and owners of The Bullworker 90™ Course, The TRISO 90™ Course, The ISO 90™ Course, and all other courses/books, publications on video, audio, and in print, together with the courses, and websites, owned, originated, and created by the copyright holders and the ISOfitness™ and TWiEA™ team, including, but not limited to all books, courses, and people mentioned in paragraph 1 of this section, accept no responsibility whatsoever for any injury, harm, damage, illness, harm, damage to property, or any other negative health-related condition which may occur as a direct, or indirect result of following these courses, recommendations, suggestions, diagrams, pictures, videos, or while performing any exercises in these or any related other related material/publication/s.

For additional general information, we also recommend that you check reputable accredited medical advice sites such as the two listed here. The National Health Service in the United Kingdom, online at: https://www.nhs.uk/Livewell/fitness/pages/physical-activity-guidelines-for-adults.aspx

In the USA, The Mayo Clinic online: http://www.mayoclinic.org/healthy-lifestyle/fitness/in-depth/exercise/art-20047414

Introduction, Precautions and Thanks

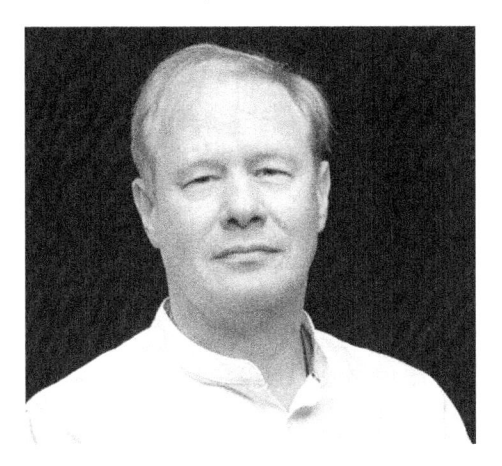

Introduction by Ajarn Stuart Hurst

After over 43 years in martial arts and in the fitness industry I have trained and exercised in many ways and found that each of them has a benefit in some way. Isometric exercise is the only system that I can take with me everywhere I go since it can be based on self-resistance. I first discovered isometric exercise many years ago when I researched the, at the time, not-so-famous Bruce Lee. I was amazed to learn how he developed his speed and power using just self-resistance, pitting one body part against another body part. This inspired me to find out more about the system, but back then it was not so easy. Over the years isometric exercise had become lost among all the gadgets and gizmos of the martial arts and wider exercise world. Bruce Lee said in a comment in an old American magazine that using yourself against yourself as a source of exercise resistance will always be the best because you are the toughest opponent you will ever face. I think that this applies perfectly to isometric exercise. So, when I am away somewhere travelling around the world filming or teaching, I perform isometric exercises regularly no matter where I am. After reading the pre-published first draft of this book I found out not only the reason why this form of exercise works so well but also about the many ways to perform isometric exercises. To be a great fighter, and/or teacher, and/or master, you have to be open to learning new things to make you continue your growth to become better. Now I am learning new things about isometric exercise, and I am also adapting this form of training into my teaching too.

MUAY THAI
The Art of Eight Limbs
The Science of Nine

Ajarn Stuart Hurst
World-Wide Copyright ©

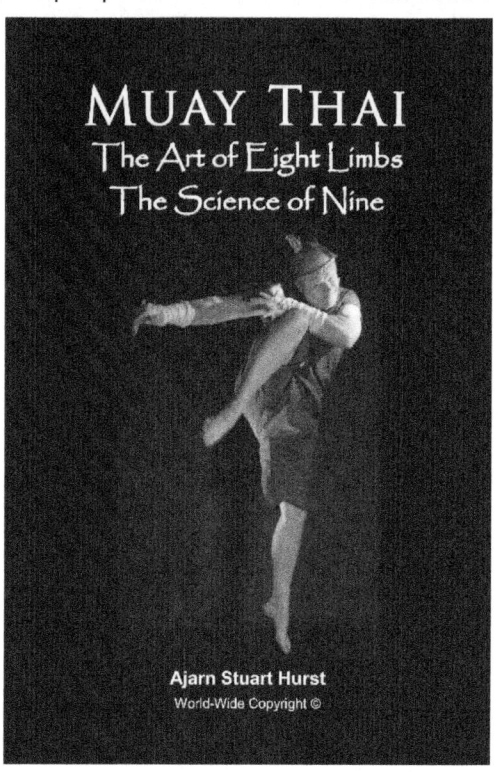

The definitive book of Muay Thai by Ajarn Stuart Hurst is available on Amazon and in all good Bookshops

MediaVision International

Ajarn Stuart Hurst, Muay Thai Champion and Master.

13

Strength and Fitness by Ajarn Sandy Holt

I have always been a massive fan of self-resisted and bodyweight-only exercises, and I practice them daily. Being strong and fit in a practical way is extremely beneficial to all martial artists. We need great strength fitness without massive muscle bulk, self-resisted and bodyweight-only exercises develop that better than anything else. This training has helped me to gain the World Record for 1 Minute Push-ups, with 132 Push-ups completed in 60 Seconds, and I came second in the World Record competition for performing the most Push-ups in 1 hour with 3,952 Push-ups. I have spent a lifetime training in Muay Thai and started training with Grandmaster Sken Kaewpadung in 1977. I was honoured to become the Double British Lightweight Thai Boxing Champion, the European Super-Featherweight Muay Thai Champion, and in 2018 to be awarded the title of Master.

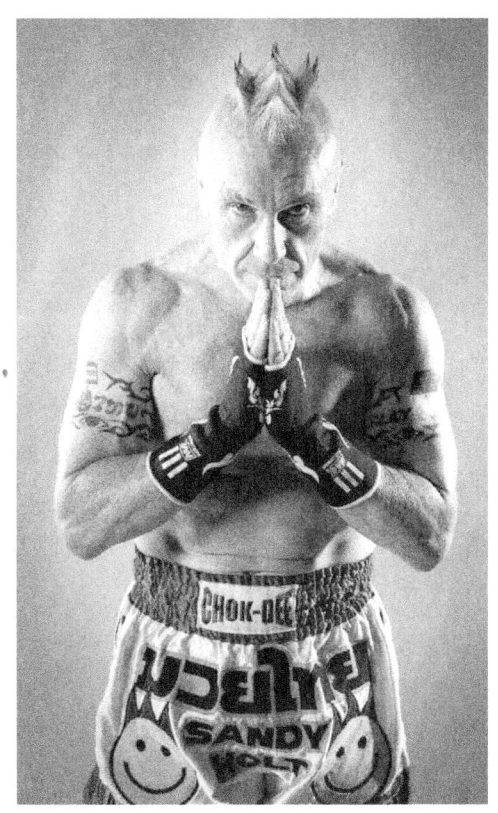

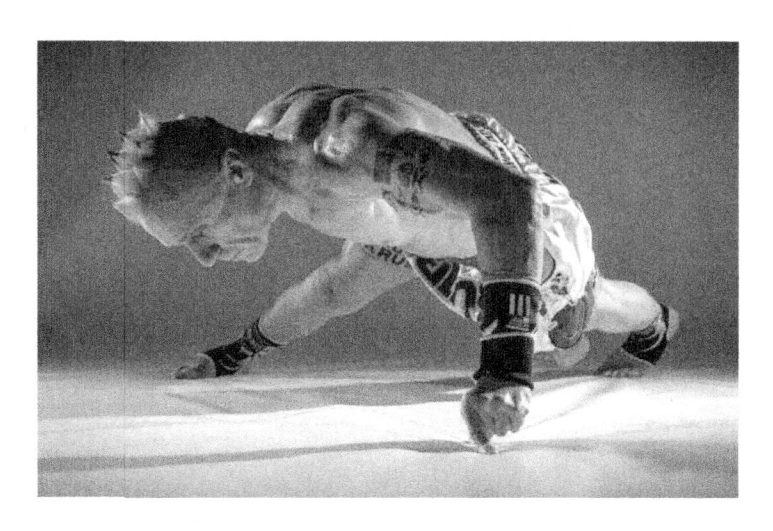

Two-Finger Push-ups
by World Record Holder Ajarn Sandy Holt
Bolton Thai Boxing Club, England.
http://thaiboxing.co.uk/

Special Precautions

Isometric exercise is not about the equipment you use, it is about the technique/s you apply. Too many people focus on the equipment as the all-important thing, and in doing so they miss out on the key elements of the system.

To this end, we have chosen to demonstrate the exercise resources in this book with our model, Marc Knowles, using nothing more than a sturdy readily available martial arts belt.

The fact is that anything could be used as a tool to perform an isometric exercise. It could be a martial arts belt as demonstrated in this book, strong climbing rope, webbing, climbers daisy chains, a Bullworker®, Steel Bow®, or Iso-Bow®, everyday immovable objects such as walls, doors and pillars etc., or by simply pitting one of your limbs against another limb.

In the true spirit of the martial arts, no isometric exercise equipment is better or worse, stronger, or weaker, they are all merely different. It is all about the person using it, their courage, strength, and applied determination that makes the real difference. However, using a piece of equipment such as an Iso-Bow® with a comfy handgrip does make performing isometric exercises much more comfortable and enjoyable to perform.

Never be afraid to experiment and try new things, but always think of safety first in everything that you do. When performing isometric exercises using a martial arts belt, or anything else for that matter, always be aware that it might slip at any moment without warning or notice.

Therefore, consider all this and plan ahead to avoid accidents that might injure you, and anyone standing near you while you exercise if the belt slips inadvertently and whips out to catch them.

Special Thanks

I would like to say a special thank you to my teachers, training partners and good friends I am about to mention. I have known all these remarkable people for most of my life, and you have all been an inspiration to me.

in no particular order, Ajarn Stuart Hurst, Sifu George Taylor, Sifu Danny Connor, Master John D. Robertson, Sensei Marc Knowles, Sensei Jacob Haynes, Dr Peter Lewis, Grandmaster Sken Kaewpadung, Grandmaster

Chinawut Sirisompan, Grandmaster Thohsaphol Sitiwatjana, Master Steve Powell, Pak Mei Grandmaster John Blackledge, Sifu Colin Oakham, Ajarn Sandy Holt, Kru Tony Moore, Master John Carrigan, Sensei Terry O'Neill.

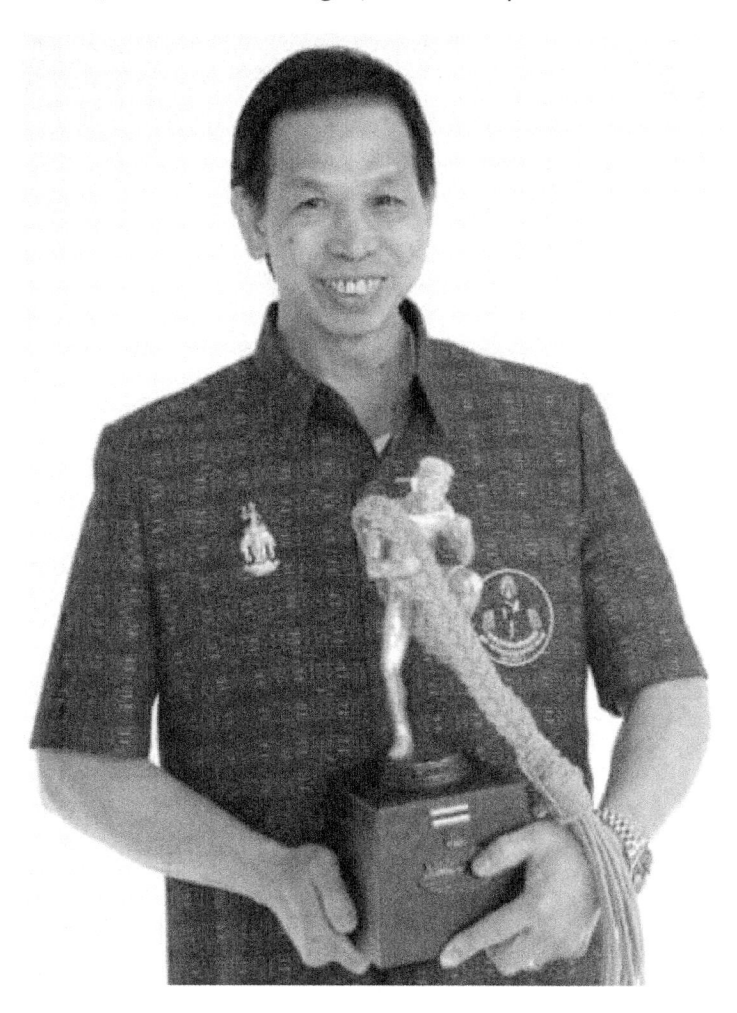

My Own Thai Master, Grandmaster Sken Kaewpadung
Grandmaster Sken Academy, Gloucestershire, England.
https://www.mastersken.com/

Chapter 1:
Isometrics, the Martial Arts and Bruce Lee

Isometric exercise and martial arts have been interlinked since people first began studying how to fight and how to improve their strength and fighting skills through training. The documented origins of isometric exercise can be traced back to around 4,000 years BC.

Interestingly, evidence supporting this begins to appear in both the Near East and the Far East almost simultaneously. However, it was the development of the more organised systems of martial arts in the Far East which brought along with it the accepted conditioning methods that became associated with each of the arts.

As the various systems of fighting evolved into the more formal structure of modern martial arts. students who were being trained were expected to assume extreme stance positions and hold them for longer periods of time to develop greater strength, fitness, and stamina.

We now refer to these as endurance isometric exercises, and since there was no such thing as exercise science to test, measure and quantify more precise forms of training. The rationale behind it all was that the longer one could hold an extreme stance or something heavy, or both, then the stronger the student would become. Through simple trial, error, and observation this type of training seemed to be particularly good at building strength, endurance, and fitness, so, over time, it gradually began to increase in popularity and eventually permeated into other martial art disciplines.

As the martial art systems developed and spread, it was not long before most, if not all, styles of martial arts began to use some form of isometric exercise as a means of conditioning students.

Obviously, the same martial arts included other style-specific methods of physical conditioning and calisthenic exercises. However, it was the isometric exercise, or 'statics' as they were known in those days, that delivered the best results.

As the various martial arts systems in China and then Japan matured, evolved, and developed into the more formal styles we know today, endurance isometrics typically became an integral part of the training system of most of the systems. Perhaps the most common type of endurance isometric employed by all systems of martial arts is when a certain combat position, and/or a training object, is held in what is generally a mechanically disadvantageous position for extended periods of time.

In the Japanese language, the term "hojo undō" means "supplementary exercises" which refers to specific conditioning methods for various styles of Karate, especially in Gōjū-ryū Karate. This system of martial arts clearly embraces and incorporates isometric exercise at the core of the system, together with other traditional callisthenics and resistance training exercises. One way of training is using Chikara Ishi, or strength stones, and more specifically the Chi-Ishi. These are basically weighted levers or mallets made of stone and/or concrete weights that are attached to a wooden pole of various lengths and thicknesses.

Karate practitioners using the Chi-Ishi would often assume difficult stances while holding the Chi-Ishi in place for long periods of time. They would also perform movements such as Kata while holding the Chi-Ishi in an endurance isometric exercise position. As all martial arts practitioners will know, Kata is a Japanese word describing precise patterns of movements simulating attack and defence techniques. It originated from the practice of paired attack and defence drills by ancient Chinese martial artists, with Kata/forms evolving as solo techniques containing concentrated sequences of movements.

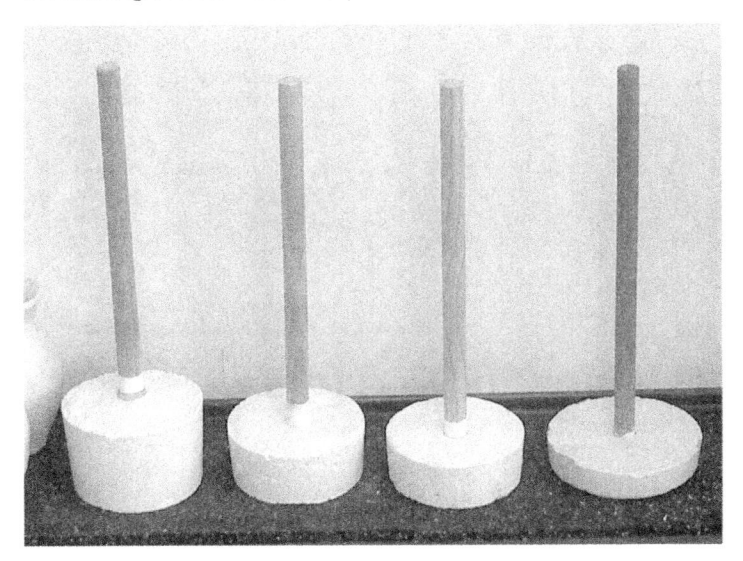

Chi Ishi Strength Stone Weights – Source: Kurmis

The wooden pole length of a Chi-Ishi would typically be between 18 and 20 inches long with a weight of some form attached only at one end. A typical martial arts club would have a selection of different Chi-Ishi weights ranging from light to heavy. Frequently, a heavy Chi-Ishi would be held for long periods by a Karateka, or a student of Karate, in a "horse stance" with the feet apart and knees bent in a semi-squat position as if they were riding a horse. It would also be often used held in the forward stance position, which is basically a leg lunge. The lighter Chi-Ishi would typically be used by gripping the pole handle as far away from the weighted end as the user's strength would allow, and then held for extended time periods in various positions away from the body. The Chi-Ishi would be used in movement-based exercises too.

The Ishi sashi, or stone lock, is another martial arts training tool that is used either for isometric or callisthenic exercises or a combination of the two. The Tetsu Ishi, or iron lock, is the metal version of essentially the same device. These resistance training tools are Chinese in origin and were later adopted by the Okinawan styles of Japanese Karate. These devices are basically what we call kettlebells today, and anyone familiar with that piece of equipment might already be able to guess how they were used in martial arts training. They vary in weight in typical increments of 5 lbs, and a

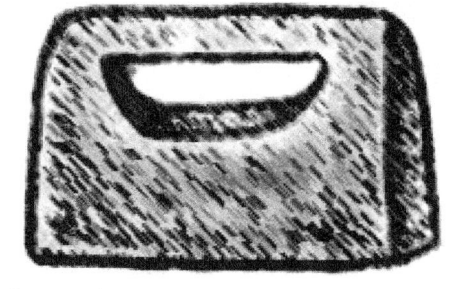

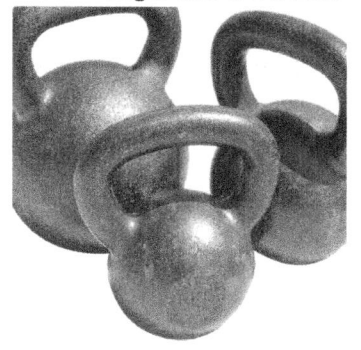

Ishi Sashi AKA the Kettlebell – Source: GiryaGirl

good martial arts club will have a comprehensive selection of them to choose from.

The Ishi Sashi, or kettlebells, are preferred exercise tools because many consider them to allow the various combat moves of the martial arts to be more closely mimicked. The heavier Ishi Sashi, AKA kettlebells, are frequently used to perform endurance isometric exercises as well as callisthenics. Interestingly, the Ishi Sashi is remarkably similar to the ancient Greek halteres dumbbell/kettlebell design.

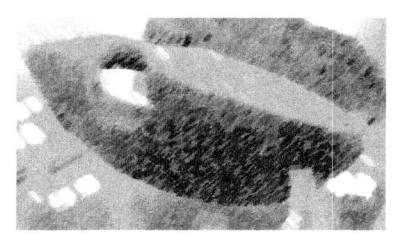

Ancient Greek Haltares

When it comes to traditional martial arts and endurance isometrics, no section would be complete without including the Nigiri game. The Nigiri game, or gripping jars, are traditional earthenware jars of various weights. Typically, they would be about 1 foot high,

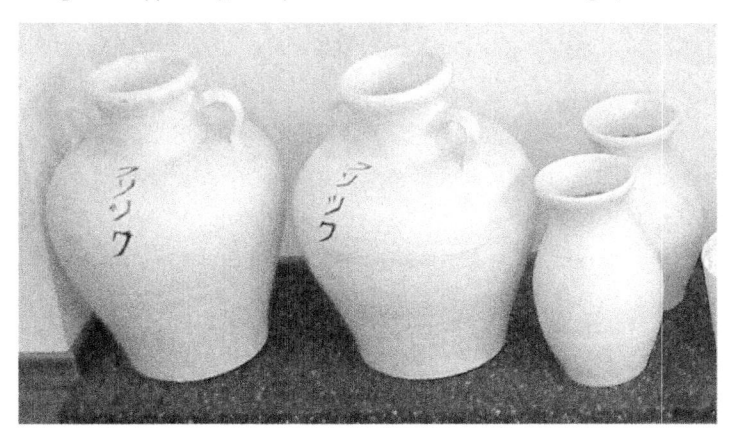

Nigiri Game Jars of Various Weights – Source: Kurmis

30.48cm, and be between 3 ½ inches, 8.89cm, and 4 ½ inches, 11.43cm, across the rim, and they would have a rim-lip of approximately ½ an inch, 1.27cm, to ¾ of an inch, 1.90cm.

The martial arts practitioners would hold, at arm's length hanging down, one jar in each hand by the lipped rim using only the fingers. Then, the martial artist would move in various ways and assume various stances while performing endurance isometric exercises for the fingers, forearms, arms, shoulders, trapezius, and neck muscles. Other muscles such as the legs, upper and lower back, chest, and core muscles would also benefit. As the martial artist grew in strength, then they would simply move up to the next weight of jar to perform the same exercises. Naturally, this form of progressive resistance would increase the intensity applied in the isometric portion of each exercise or exercise combination.

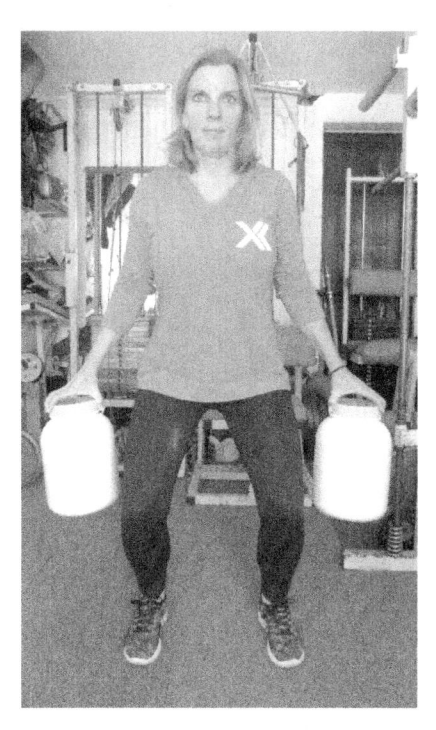

Another basic exercise that is frequently performed is to carry the jars as far as possible while being gripped only by the fingers around the rim. This exercise is more commonly known as "the farmers walk" or "carry" which is typically used in modern strength competitions. Many use sand or small stones in the jars, while others prefer to use water to provide the weight. Some believe that even though using water in the jars might sometimes make the weight lighter than if stones or sand were used, the constant movement of the water and the instability it provides as it shifts and settles, add a new and very challenging dimension to the training.

It was almost certainly the legendary Bruce Lee who cemented the modern cultural link between martial arts and isometric exercise. Bruce Lee was an exercise fanatic and made it one of his life goals to research and evaluate every type of exercise available. Even when he was resting or working in his office, his close friends and aides reported that Bruce would hook himself up to an Electrical Muscle Stimulation (EMS) machine to continue exercising his muscles outside of the gym. With an EMS machine, impulses are generated by a device and are delivered through electrodes on the skin near the muscles one wished to be stimulated like they are when exercised. Electrode pads adhere to the skin so the

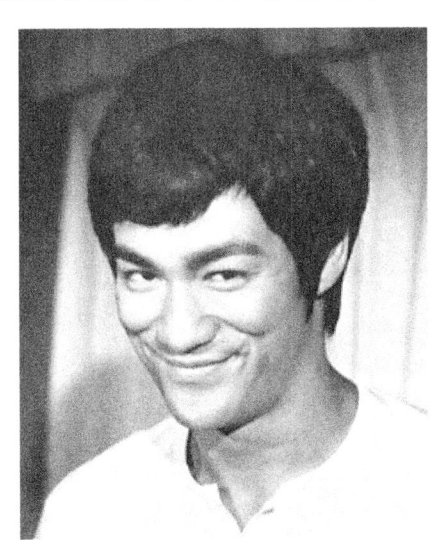

Bruce Lee

impulses generated by the machine can be delivered to mimic the action potential that comes from the central nervous system causing the muscles to contract. This sort of behaviour only goes to show just how keen Bruce Lee was when it came to exercise and efficiency.

Bruce Lee's love of efficiency and using only what worked well in all things was reflected in his system of martial arts. Bruce developed his own system by studying and combining only the most efficient and practical elements from many different martial arts. He called his system Jeet Kune Do, which in Cantonese means "The way of the intercepting fist" and is abbreviated simply as JKD. This is a hybrid system founded the system on July 9, 1967. Bruce referred to it as being "non-classical" which essentially made it a formless form of Kung Fu. In developing JKD, if the analysis showed Bruce that a traditional martial arts system incorporated wasted movements, attacks, defences, or rituals, then they would be removed so that the essence of what remained was only the most efficient elements of the art.

Therefore, it should be no surprise to anyone that Bruce Lee loved isometric exercise so much because it worked so efficiently. Bruce soon found that isometric exercise was one of the best ways to build great strength, endurance, fitness, and muscle power. More importantly, it did not build the bulky bodybuilder type of muscle bulk, but rather the rock-solid muscle and strength which was, without doubt, the most practical for all forms of martial arts combat. Big, bulky bodybuilder-style muscles have always been the enemy of combat sports. There is a critical mass point where muscle size and strength meet what is fighting-efficient, and bulky bodybuilder-style muscles have never worked well in practice.

Bruce Lee was famous for performing what I call inertia isometrics, such as lifting barbells or smith machine bars into positions to perform isometric exercises. Technically, Inertia is the resistance of a physical object to a change in its velocity. In other words, the mass of a barbell in a gym provides resistance to the person lifting it as exercise. This means that when this heavy object is lifted into a position to perform an isometric exercise, the elements of mass and inertia place a much greater overall demand on many more muscles in the body than would otherwise be activated by simply performing limb-against-limb resisted isometric exercises. Gymnastic-Style Bodyweight only and Biomechanically Disadvantaged style (GSBBD) isometric exercises also fall into the inertia isometrics category.

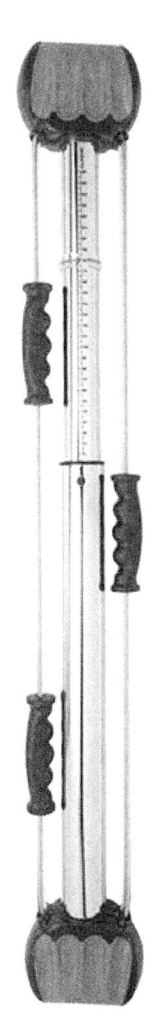

When it came to Bruce's love of all things that were practical and efficient, his favourite isometric exercise tool was almost certainly the legendary Bullworker®. The Bullworker® was developed in the 1960s by the famous German exercise science expert, Gert F. Kölbel. The invention of the Bullworker® instantly revolutionised the world of home exercise because it enabled almost anyone to train virtually every major muscle of the body intensely, and yet without the need for a commercial gymnasium. Since the Bullworker® delivered real results that people could see and feel within a comparatively short time, it soon became a "must-have" device for anyone serious about excelling at their chosen sport. Bruce Lee soon recognised the power and potential of what was effectively an amazing portable multi-gym.

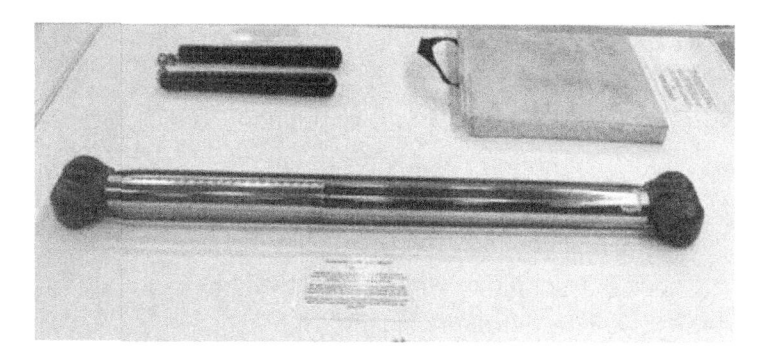

Bruce Lee's Bullworker®, Nunchaku, and Makiwara.

The invention of the Bullworker® by Gert F. Kölbel as a combined isometric and isotonic device was, by and large, inspired by the results of a 5-year scientific study into the effectiveness of isometric exercise at the world-famous Max Plank Institute in Dortmund, Germany.

Between 1953 and 1958, one of the most extensive research studies ever undertaken was commissioned into isometric exercise science. These experiments are now considered by many to be the original "gold standard" of all exercise studies. The results of this were first made public knowledge in the ground-breaking book, "The Physiology of Strength," by Dr Theodor Hettinger - Research Fellow at the Max Plank Institute.

During that 5-year research period, Dr Hettinger and Dr Muller performed over 5,500 experiments on volunteers from all walks of life, and at every level of strength, fitness, and athletic ability. The test subjects even included serious strength athletes and middle-aged, overweight, and unfit people of both sexes. Perhaps what surprised people the most was how dramatic and impressive the results were gained from performing simple isometric exercises. Also, because the same or extremely similar results were easily repeatable time and time again, it made the data gathered from the experiments extremely reliable.

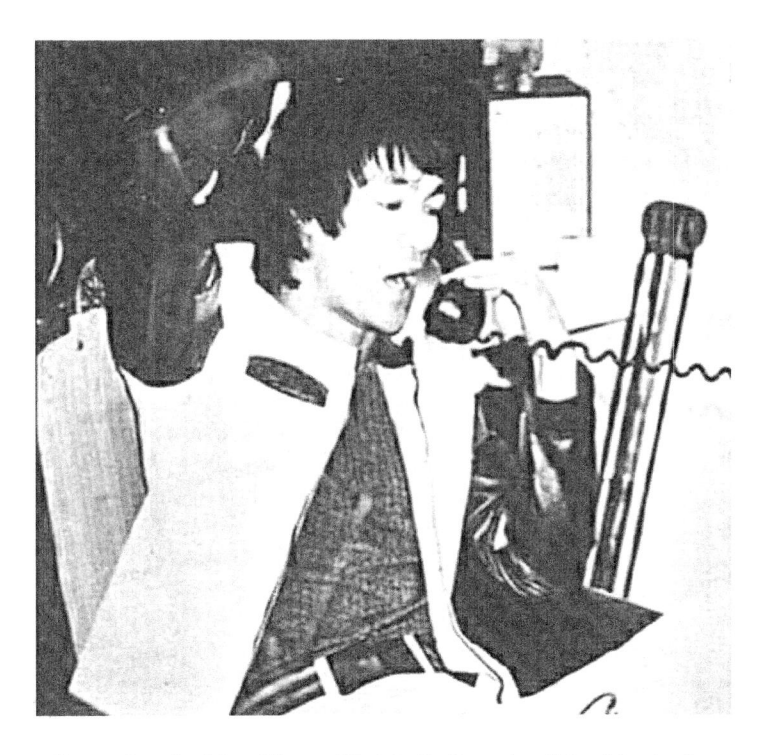

Bruce Lee in his office with his Bullworker® by his desk.

The conclusions of the study proved beyond doubt that when compared to traditional isotonic exercise methods, isometric exercise was superior in developing great strength and muscle size in minimum time. It also proved that the isometric system delivered these results much faster and with far less exercise than traditional resistance training methods.

Therefore, it should be of no surprise then why Bruce Lee loved both the isometric exercises system and his Bullworker®. To Bruce, the combination of the two was unbeatable as a method of physical conditioning to attain optimum strength, power, and combat readiness. More importantly, Bruce loved that he could take his Bullworker® with him everywhere he went, and he was famous for maintaining his regular workout sessions no matter where he was, or what he was doing. For Bruce Lee, it was all about fitness without frontiers or restrictions.

Today, it is unfortunate that isometric exercise has become slightly less mainstream and much more marginalised. The professional mainstream image of isometric exercise has not been helped by social media forums. These places have become a breeding ground for the occasional self-professed 'guru' and/or isometric 'sage' to appear, the whacky idea merchants, and the keyboard warriors whom all believe that they are isometric exercise experts, usually for no other reason than the fact that they own an isometric exercise device.

This sort of thing only serves to play right into the hands of all those who wish to marginalise isometric exercise and tarnish its overall image to suit their own ends.

Typically, this is purely driven because of the commercial interests of gym owners and personal trainers who do not really want the general public to know that they could easily substitute many expensive and time-consuming gym sessions for fast, effective, and very inexpensive isometrics.

The fact is that it should never be an either/or scenario when it comes to exercise choice. All techniques and systems have merit and value if performed correctly. Isometric exercise is every bit as good as traditional callisthenic exercise, with both techniques having certain advantages and disadvantages when compared. In keeping with the spirit of the martial arts, nothing is better or worse, stronger, or weaker, they are merely different and have equal merit.

Fortunately, isometric exercise is still very much alive, well, and typically still highly revered in almost all martial arts clubs around the world.

The big difference between isometric exercise today and when science first began to thoroughly research it is that we now know much more about the science behind it and the range of isometric exercise techniques that have enormous value.

This means that the modern martial arts instructor is no longer restricted to simply using and coaching endurance isometric techniques. Instead, they have a much wider range of isometric exercise techniques available to them. We will explain more about some of these in a later section.

I decided to write this book to combine my lifelong study and practice of several martial arts systems with my other life-long study of exercise science, and in particular isometric exercise. No matter what type of martial art is practised, I wanted both martial arts instructors and students alike to have access to a range of practical exercises, together with enough knowledge of isometric exercise science to help them improve their overall fighting skills through having greater overall strength and martial arts 'firepower' without the impractical muscle bulk that could easily slow them down.

TWiEA, The World Isometric Exercise Association has also embraced the link between martial arts and isometric exercise. TWiEA now offers an approved isometric exercise instructor training course for exercise professionals and martial artists who want to learn the safest and most efficient isometric exercise techniques and how to teach them.

Isometric exercise has come a long way from its humble beginnings thousands of years ago. Today, it is a proven, powerful science-based exercise system that delivers more results in less time and with less exercise than traditional exercise systems. For the modern martial artist, the future is bright, the future is Isometric Power Exercises for Martial Arts.

Chapter 2:
Exercise Science Overview

In this section, we will give a user-friendly overview of exercise science together with the features and benefits of various exercise techniques and concepts. For those who want more in-depth information about the science of isometric exercise and health and fitness in general, then we suggest that you also read our books The ISOmetric Bible™ and The 70 Second Difference™ books. Both are available on Amazon.

The Basic Types of Resistance Exercise

All muscle training falls into between two or three specific categories, depending upon how you break them down. In the most basic form, there are two types, either contraction with movement, or contraction without movement. Breaking them down a step further there become three categories, with one being isotonic, another isokinetic. Last but certainly not least, is isometric.

Isotonic training is all about movement with muscle shortening and lengthening during the lifting and lowering phases of the exercise. We know that the isotonic category can be broken down further into three parts. One part is the concentric contraction, which is the lifting phase of an exercise when the muscles shorten. Another is the eccentric phase which is the lowering part of an exercise when the muscles lengthen.

Lastly in this isotonic category is the isokinetic contraction. This is where the muscle changes in length during both the concentric and eccentric phases of the contraction, however, the velocity remains constant no matter how much force is applied during the exercises.

Then comes the isometric category. With an isometric exercise, there is no movement whatsoever. To help you envision this, I will take a random weight training or freehand callisthenic exercise such as a chest press because it can be performed either with movement OR without movement, as an isometric exercise.

For example, a barbell, a machine, or your bodyweight can be lifted and lowered to perform an exercise such as a barbell curl, this is called, isotonic exercise, callisthenics or simply exercise with movement.

To perform the same or similar exercise isometrically you would attempt to perform the same or similar biomechanically correct actions of a barbell curl, however, at a certain point, or points if multiple exercise points were being used, the curling movement would stop because an immovable object point had been reached.

At that point or points, you would apply an increasing level of intensity until you reach the desired target level as you attempt to perform the curling exercise against the immovable object.

At the desired isometric exercise point, a constant force is applied against the immovable object for 7 seconds which is the optimum isometric exercise time. The ideal basic isometric exercise point for general exercise is roughly at the mid-point when your muscles reach a stalemate working against each other or an immovable object. This is called a Standard isometric Contraction.

The harder you engage your muscles as you try to break the stalemate by lifting, pushing, or pulling, then the stronger your muscles become. In doing so, you engage many more muscle fibres than normal as you attempt to move the immovable object and perform the curling exercise action.

Doors, desks, chairs, walls, and many other everyday items work well as immovable objects BUT the easiest and most used immovable object is typically yourself.

Isometric Overview

As you now know, isometric exercise does not involve any movement. Instead, the joint angle and the muscle length do not change during contraction. You also now know that 7 seconds is now regarded as the optimum time to perform an isometric exercise.

However, almost everyone when exercising tends to count the exercise elapsed time much faster than real elapsed time. This means that it is easy not to reach the magic 7 seconds of the optimum isometric exercise time. Therefore, we always suggest aiming to perform the exercise for 10 seconds to ensure that the 7-second target is always reached even when under the stress of performing intense exercise.

Isometric exercise has been extensively scientifically researched and has been proven time and again to be a highly efficient way to build great strength and grow muscle. In fact, isometric exercise is probably one of the most thoroughly researched of all exercise systems.

However, it also remains one of the most misunderstood systems of exercise. This is almost certainly through fear, professional ignorance, and purely financial reasons.

Several different techniques can be used in the isometric exercise system. Most of these techniques are highly advanced for use by competitive athletes, competitive martial arts practitioners, strength athletes and bodybuilders. Therefore, they have no application as part of a general isometric exercise session for the average person who simply wants to get generally stronger and fitter.

However, purely out of interest I will list them here, and in case any fitness enthusiasts, athletes or bodybuilders read this book and wish to try them. They are described in greater detail in our book called The Isometric Bible which is available on Amazon and in good bookstores. The most common and advanced isometric exercise techniques include the following:

- Standard Isometric Contraction
- Yielding Isometric Contraction
- Maximum Duration Isometrics
- Oscillatory Isometrics
- Impact Absorption Isometrics
- Explosive Isometrics, AKA: Ballistic Isometrics
- Static-Dynamic Isometric
- Isometric Contrast
- Functional Isometrics
- TRISOmetrics™

There are more than enough isometric exercises that can be performed without any equipment whatsoever to allow a total body workout routine to be completed relatively easily. These will typically be self-resisted isometric exercises, which are excellent. However, by using only minimal readily available equipment such as walking poles, golf clubs, martial arts belts, climbing ropes, scuba diving webbing weight belts, and broom handles etc. it is possible to greatly expand the number of exercises that can be performed.

It is also perfectly possible to adapt and use other readily available items such as tow ropes, steel chains, towels, and commonly found immobile objects such as sturdy fixed barrier railings, solid walls, solid doors, door frames, or parked vehicles to perform a complete isometric exercise routine. Again, these are all excellent improvised exercise tools that allow an expanded range of highly effective isometric exercises to be performed.

Using improvised exercise tools can yield an unexpected additional benefit. This is because it allows one to focus more and apply greater concentration to each exercise. This is particularly useful for those who are either completely new to, or who are relatively new to the isometric exercise system. We will explain more about what these can be later in the book.

One of the things we love about both the isometric and self-resisted systems of exercise is that as you get stronger through exercise, then you can apply more force and intensity to your isometric or self-resisted exercises.

This, in turn, means that you can gradually increase the level of intensity you can safely apply to each exercise which will mean that the results and benefits you receive will grow in a compound way through regular daily use. This is what we call a natural Adaptive Response™ mechanism which is a useful aspect of our biology.

Isometric Exercise Science

Even until the mid-20th century, there was almost no scientific research that had been performed into the benefits of isometric exercise. We also know that before the first serious scientific research study, how people trained isometrically was typically by performing what we now call endurance isometrics.

Thankfully, isometric exercise has now been thoroughly scientifically researched and proven for several decades. I would estimate that there has probably been at least as much scientific research performed into isometric exercise as there has been into traditional resistance training.

The first major in-depth study into isometric exercise was performed at the world-famous Max Plank Institute in Dortmund, Germany. If you already have a reasonable knowledge of science, you will also know that the Max Plank Institute is a world-renowned centre of scientific excellence in many disciplines.

Between 1953 and 1958, one of the most extensive research studies was commissioned into isometric exercise science. These experiments are now considered by many to be the original gold standard of isometric exercise studies. The results were made widespread public knowledge in the resultant ground-breaking book, The Physiology of Strength, by Dr Theodor Hettinger - Research Fellow at the Max Plank

Institute. During that 5-year research period, Dr Hettinger and Dr Muller performed a widely reported, reputed 5,500 experiments, although this figure is almost certainly apocryphal because they would have had to perform a minimum of three experiments a day, every day for five years. Research suggests that the actual number of experiments performed by Hettinger and Muller was probably closer to 200, however, in wider studies at other institutions since that time, over 5,500 studies have almost certainly been completed. These were conducted on male and female volunteers from all walks of life, and at every level of strength, fitness, and athletic ability. Perhaps what surprised people the most was how dramatic and impressive the results were gained from performing isometric exercises. Also, because the same or similar results were easily repeatable it made the data gained from the experiments exceptionally reliable.

Another extremely interesting result emerged from the experiments. This was because it was not the length of time that an isometric exercise was held that produced the optimum results. Instead, it was the correct level of intensity applied for a very specific optimum time.

They found that performing only one daily isometric exercise for between only 6 and 7 seconds, and at only two-thirds of an individual's maximum effort, could increase strength by an average of up to 5% per week. By any standards, strength gains of 5% in exchange for the expenditure of only 66%, or around two-thirds of an individual's maximum capacity, is an excellent result.

Perhaps even more amazingly, they discovered that after someone has performed a single 7-second training stimulus (exercise) per day, the muscle being exercised in that same position was no longer responsive to further gains. In other words, it did not matter how many more times you exercised the same muscle in the same position, there would be no further increase in muscle growth or strength. The only way to do this was to perform another isometric exercise at a different position only the ROM (Range Of Motion) of the limb being exercised. The scientific data about this can be referenced on pages 28 to 31 of Dr Theodor Hettinger's book, The Physiology of Strength.

In 2001, Nicolas Babault PhD of the University of Burgundy, Dijon, France, led a team of scientists to research and examine how many muscle fibres were activated, and how long they remained active, during both traditional weight training and isometric training.

(The scientific research paper is published: Nicolas Babault, Michel Pousson, Yves Ballay, and Jacques Van Hoecke - Groupe Analyse du Mouvement, Unite´ de Formation et de Recherche Sciences et Techniques des Activite´s Physiques et Sportives, Universite´ de Bourgogne, BP 27877, 21078 Dijon Cedex, France.)

They discovered that when training intensely, and in near-perfect style, the levels of muscle activation during repetitions of optimum maximal weight training were between 89.7% during the concentric contraction, or when lifting a weight, and 88.3% during the eccentric contraction, or when lowering a weight. For practical purposes, an average of about 89% overall.

    The study also revealed that during the lifting, or concentric part of the exercise, the maximum intramuscular tension only lasted for between 0.25 and 0.5 seconds. Which, for practical purposes is an average of about 1/3rd of a second during each isotonic repetition.

    This is because traditional isotonic resistance exercises naturally involve movement. They also have aspects of velocity and acceleration to consider in the overall equation. "Force" is only produced for a split second, to produce a maximal contraction of the muscle fibres.

    The same research also showed that the level of muscle activation during isometric exercise was as high as 95.2% and that it lasted for the entire 7 to 10 seconds of each exercise. This is a huge increase over the 1/3rd of second muscular activation achieved during a single repetition of weight training. Therefore, based on these discoveries, then technically a single isometric exercise performed at only two-thirds of an individual's overall maximum can deliver either similar or often even better results, than the equivalent of up to 3 sets of 10 weight training repetitions in the lifting phase of the exercise.

    To explain this further I will use a typical barbell curl exercise in the lifting phase as my example, where the object of the exercise is to engage as many muscle fibres as possible in a maximum muscular contraction. Naturally, 3 sets of 10 repetitions give us an overall total of 30 repetitions. One set of 10 repetitions of the barbell curl in perfect high-intensity style produces a total maximum muscular engagement for a total of approximately 3.3 seconds. Three sets of 10 repetitions of the same exercise, a total of 30 repetitions will give a total of approximately 9.9 seconds of maximum muscular engagement, and an average of 89% muscle activation overall.

In comparison, one high-intensity isometric contraction exercise produces a maximum muscular engagement that lasts for the entire duration of the exercise. Even though the optimum time over which an isometric exercise is performed was found to be 7 seconds, this is almost always rounded up to the 10-second target number. The maximum muscular engagement will last for the entire 10 seconds of a high-intensity isometric exercise and with 95.2% muscle activation overall.

This is proof that is based entirely on scientific research that 3 sets of 10 near-perfect high-intensity curls when weight training, which takes several minutes to perform, still were not equal to the results achieved by a single 10-second high-intensity isometric curl exercise.

The Standard Isometric Contraction

The standard isometric contraction is a simple and highly effective technique. Therefore, this is the technique we will focus on for practical isometric training.

The standard isometric contraction, AKA: overcoming isometric contraction, AKA: maximum-effort isometrics, or whatever else you wish to call it, is when a muscle is applying force to push or pull against an immovable resistance. This is the most basic of all kinds of isometric exercise, and it is highly effective.

This type of isometric contraction exercise was performed during the experiments by Dr T. Hettinger and Dr E. Muller at the Max Plank Institute. It is also the technique referred to in their book The Physiology of Strength.

In a standard isometric contraction, it is theoretically possible to exert up to 100% of one's maximum capacity effort against an immovable object and then continue to hold that level of intensity throughout the exercise. This means that standard isometric contraction can be a very high-intensity exercise system.

Performing an isometric exercise against an immovable object at a certain level of intensity for a given duration of time will teach your body to recruit more muscle fibres to try to move the object. As you perform the exercise and generate as much force as possible, your CNS, or Central Nervous System, learns that it needs to activate and recruit more muscle fibres to reach the goal of moving the object.

Since this will naturally be impossible to move, the process will continue each time you exercise to make you stronger and grow more muscle. Your body mechanisms become trained to readily activate and recruit additional muscle fibres as needed when facing repeated similar challenges, which in turn, repeats the cycle more readily every time.

As we mentioned earlier, the immovable/solid object that is used can be anything that is completely solid and completely safe to use. This can be a wall, a door, a door jamb, a parked motor vehicle or anything similar. Perhaps the most common objects used to enhance everyday isometric exercise training are sturdy towels, climbing ropes, martial arts belts, scuba diving weight belts, webbing straps, golf clubs, and broom handles, etc. All the aforementioned items are excellent when used properly, and all will deliver some excellent results. More importantly, they are typically readily available for most people which makes exercising with them so much easier.

Another common way to perform isometric exercise is to do it in a self-resisted way. Self-resisted means that you push or pull against your limbs, hands, and feet, etc. For example, you might place the palms of your hands together at chest level with your hands roughly at the midpoint of your body. In that position, you would then press your hands together using your chest muscles to provide the primary driving force. Suddenly, you are performing a highly effective self-resisted isometric chest exercise!

It is possible to perform a well-balanced and highly effective self-resisted isometric workout to exercise virtually every section of the body. So, never underestimate self-resisted exercise because it can be immensely powerful indeed. Also, self-resistance exercises are an excellent way to ensure that a personal maximum resistance is used safely, and with minimum risk of injury caused by applying too much force.

The fact is that it does not matter which method is chosen. It can be isometrics performed against an immovable object, self-resisted isometrics, or a combination of the two. The most important thing is that either the object must be completely immovable through human muscle power alone, or the force of one body part must be able to completely counterbalance the force of another body part to produce a muscular stalemate.

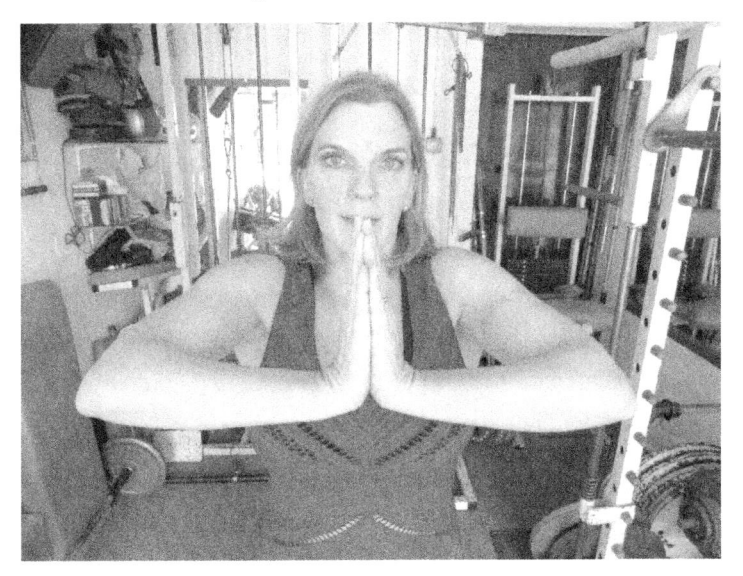

Workout Intensity

Intensity is always going to be a relative term, and it is often completely misunderstood when it is used concerning exercise. When it comes to exercising your muscles, the intensity is the % of your ability to move a resistance. Technically, an individual's highest possible level of intensity is when they reach a point of momentary failure after exerting themselves completely.

However, the important questions we need to try and find answers to are: "How hard is hard?" and "How intense is intense?" To some degree, both are very subjective things. Taking two people of roughly equal fitness, something that is intense to one person might be considered comparatively easy to the other.

Hard is a relative term, and handling 50 lbs of resistance is impossibly hard if your strength is only at the level required to lift 49 lbs. However, if you can lift 100 lbs as a maximum, then lifting 50 lbs is going to be comparatively easy.

Often, the only factors differentiating between people and the intensity level exerted, are going to be mental toughness, determination, and perception.

Therefore, to gain the greatest benefits from isometric exercise the first thing that must be learned is how to determine, with a reasonable degree of accuracy, what level of intensity is being applied to an exercise.

It is just a fact that what one person deems to be 100% of their capacity will always be quite different from another person's estimate. The accurate estimation of what one person deems to be $2/3^{rds}$ of their overall maximum intensity will also vary from person to person. The accuracy of estimation will also vary greatly between an experienced professional athlete and an absolute beginner to exercise.

Experience has taught us that most people who are new to exercise will always fall well short of accurate estimation of any given percentage. A beginner will find it more challenging to accurately estimate what $2/3^{rds}$ of their 100% maximum is when compared to a more experienced athlete. Many people might believe that they are performing at 100% capacity when they are only performing at around only 2/3rds, or even perhaps at only 50% or less of their 100% maximum.

This is because exercise is new to them, therefore, the experiences and feelings in their body which are associated with it are also new. They simply have no common frame of reference when it comes to calculating/estimating their level of physical exertion.

The human brain has a built-in mechanism that helps to protect the body and prevent it from performing physical activity to such a level that could cause serious damage or even death. This is the mechanism that makes your brain tell you to stop exercising when it begins to get tough, and the feeling of wanting to stop exercising only increases as you continue to push yourself harder to do more. This is all despite the biological fact that you are physically capable of doing much more than is being suggested by the messages you are receiving from yourself.

Over time, the brain of people who exercise regularly, and especially to a high level of intensity, will naturally adjust, and reposition this built-in safety margin. This means that the brain of an experienced high-level athlete does not "tell" them to stop an exercise until the level of intensity is much higher than it would be for a beginner.

Therefore, when it comes to exercise, how is it possible to subjectively quantify, and then impart appropriate levels of recommended intensity? This problem is made even more challenging when one considers the fact that accurately translating and subjectively assessing various levels of intensity will, to some degree, always be subjective to every individual.

If you were to train as hard as humanly possible, with near 100% maximum intensity which involves super-strict form, and training to complete failure and beyond, then you simply cannot train for a long time. It is just physiologically impossible. Physics and biology are quite simple in this respect.

The intensity of your workout is directly proportional to the length of time that you are physically able to perform your workout. The harder and more intensely you exercise, then the shorter time that you will be physically able to perform the exercise.

Make no mistake, performing a 7-second isometric exercise while exerting close to your personal 100% maximum physical capacity is completely and utterly exhausting, even for a professional athlete.

What does all this mean when it comes to accurately communicating to others various levels of exercise intensity, especially when there is no professional coach or expensive measuring equipment at hand?

Research clearly shows that almost everyone will stop exercising long before they are in any danger of becoming seriously fatigued. Most people will *think* they are achieving a much higher level of intensity than they would if they were only a little more mentally resilient.

This does not mean that people should suddenly begin pushing themselves beyond their physical limits, which would be a stupid thing to do. However, it does mean that most people who enjoy a higher-than-average level of mental resilience and determination, as well as being in physically good condition, can push themselves much harder than they might think. If anyone ever feels "genuine" strain or fatigue to the point of becoming injured, then they should stop exercising immediately.

Even without the aid of a professional coach to monitor, encourage you and measure your intensity and progress with specialist equipment, the tips we have outlined in this section will help you to get the most out of every workout. It is also worth remembering that if you cheat, then the only person who loses is "you."

Technically, How Does a Muscle Grow?

How does a muscle grow? This is one of the most common questions asked concerning fitness and exercise in general. However, it is also one of the most misunderstood concepts, even amongst fitness professionals and personal trainers. To see for yourself just how uninformed or badly informed some people are, simply join one or two of the social media groups online so you can read some of the absolute drivel posted by 'keyboard warriors' who purport to be 'experts' on the subject. Alarmingly, many of these people seem to have developed a hardcore following, which to the science-based professional is like watching 'fools leading other fools' on a wild goose chase.

So, back to the key question which is, how does a muscle grow? To explain this, we must examine three concepts, which are: 1) muscle growth through increases in the volume/size of myofibrils inside the muscles, which is commonly termed myofibrillar hypertrophy. 2) hyperplasia, which is when there is an increase in the number of muscle cells/fibres. 3) sarcoplasmic growth which is all about increasing the fluid content.

When it comes to the subject of exercise, the muscles you wish to grow must be challenged with a workload that is greater than they can currently accommodate. In other words, an exercise that is intense enough to stimulate growth. This stimulus can come from any source such as lifting a heavy object, weight training, isometrics, compressing a spring in a device such as a Bullworker™, or through self-resistance either hand to hand or limb to limb or using an Iso-Bow™ etc.

This process creates trauma to the muscle fibres which disrupts the muscle cell organelles. This then triggers other cells outside the muscle fibres to greatly increase in numbers at and around the point of the trauma to repair the damage. The process of repair involves a fusion of cells. This, in turn, causes the cross-sectional area of the muscle fibre to increase because the muscle cell myofibrils increase in both size and quantity. This process is more commonly known as hypertrophy. Since this process increases the number of cellular nuclei the muscle fibres generate more myosin and actin. These are contractile protein myofilaments which in turn help to make the muscle stronger.

This is the basis of what is more commonly known as myofibril muscle growth. In addition to this, there is also probably a process called hyperplasia which takes place. I use the term, 'probably' because this concept is extremely controversial for many reasons. One of the key problems is that evidence of this in human beings is lacking, whereas there is a mass of evidence supporting hyperplasia in mice and other animals.

Hypertrophy is the increase in the size of the existing muscle fibres to accommodate the increased demands placed upon them through intense exercise. Hyperplasia, concerning skeletal muscle growth, is the increase in the number of muscle fibres which in turn will also increase the cross-sectional area of a muscle.

Despite there being a lack of evidence supporting hyperplasia in human beings, logic supports the process taking place. This is because of a theory known as Nuclear Domain Theory. This states that the nucleus of a cell (a muscle cell in this instance) is only able to control a finite area of cellular space. It is thought that satellite cells donate their nuclei to the muscle cell until a certain point is reached whereby this can no longer take place. Beyond a certain limit, and through continued intense training, the cell must eventually divide to create two cells instead of the former single cell. When this happens, the entire hypertrophy process starts over once again. This probably means that most of the muscle growth is almost certainly caused by hypertrophy, and a much smaller percentage can be attributed to hyperplasia at any given point in the muscle stimulus/growth process.

Finally, there is a subject of sarcoplasmic muscle growth to address. Sarcoplasmic muscle growth is the increase in the volume of sarcoplasmic fluid in the muscle cell. These are the fluid and energy resources surrounding the myofibrils in your muscles containing mostly glycogen together with other elements including creatine, ATP, and water etc.

To clarify, glycogen is simply a type of sugar that serves as a form of energy. It is deposited in bodily tissues as a store of carbohydrates, and it is the body's main form of storage for the sugar, glucose. Glycogen is stored in two main places in the body, one being the liver, and the other being the muscles.

More importantly, glycogen is the body's secondary source of long-term energy storage, with the primary energy storage source being fat. When glycogen is in the muscles, it is converted into glucose for use as energy when performing sports etc., and glycogen stored in the liver is converted into glucose for use as energy throughout the body, and in the central nervous system.

Therefore, sarcoplasmic growth increases muscle volume, but this increase is not in functional strength mass since it does not increase the number of muscle fibres. It is like 'the pump', in that it is an increase in the size and shape of the muscle through the muscle holding an increased amount of fluid.

Rest Time Between Exercises

Naturally, the rest time taken between exercises during a workout is quite different from the rest and recovery needed to recover and allow your body to positively respond to the stimulus generated by exercise.

If you keep the rest time between exercises brief enough, then the workout routine itself will give you an excellent cardiovascular workout, and this is what we recommend that you ultimately aim for. If you are already very fit, then we would recommend that instead of performing the optional cardio routine you simply put more effort and intensity into each isometric exercise. At the same time, aim to keep the rest time between those exercises as brief as possible. This approach will help you work towards being able to perform each exercise so that it has an Ultra-High Intensity Ultra-Short Burst™ effect, which will greatly improve your overall fitness level, and boost your Base Metabolic Rate or BMR.

However, if you are not already fit, then to begin with you may wish to simply allow each isometric exercise to deliver all the cardio you need as you gradually build up your levels of fitness and endurance. Eventually, you will soon increase your level of fitness to a point where you can begin to gradually reduce the rest time between each exercise to a minimum point that works best for you.

Once you have learned how to fully engage the muscles during each exercise with sufficient intensity, and at the same time, you have learned how to breathe fully, deeply, and naturally throughout each exercise. At the same time, you should be keeping the rest time between exercises to a minimum because this combination will have an excellent and beneficial cardiovascular effect.

Dynamic Flexation™

Dynamic Flexation™ is a technique we devised to help ensure that we gained maximum benefit from the isometric portion of our exercise regimens. I will recap and briefly summarise the Dynamic Flexation™ technique as originally laid out in "The 70 Second Difference™" book.

We always recommend that everyone who performs any kind of resistance exercise practices some form of Dynamic Flexation™ before performing any exercise. This will help to ensure that all muscles, tendons, ligaments, joints, and your spine have become naturally and properly engaged in the correct biomechanical exercise position.

We would never recommend that as soon as you assume any exercise position you suddenly apply maximum power and intensity right away. This is unless you are a very experienced athlete, or unless you are training with a qualified coach to perform a certain type of isometric exercise to develop extra power such as a static-dynamic or explosive/ballistic isometric technique. Instead, we recommend that you always breathe naturally as you gradually flex and engage your muscles and joints into performing the exercise.

To perform Dynamic Flexation™ you gradually flex your grip and the muscles you are about to exercise while applying an increasing level of intensity immediately before performing the exercise. The exercise is then performed, and to disengage from the exercise we recommend reversing the Dynamic Flexation™ engagement process.

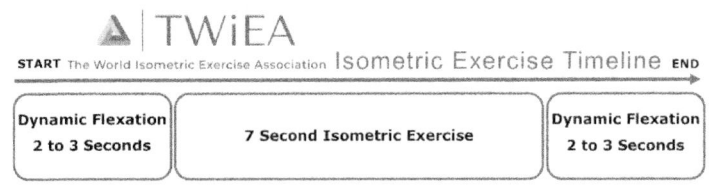

▲ | TWiEA

START The World Isometric Exercise Association Isometric Exercise Timeline **END**

| Dynamic Flexation 2 to 3 Seconds | 7 Second Isometric Exercise | Dynamic Flexation 2 to 3 Seconds |

Our preference is to apply tension and intensity to the exercise gradually through Dynamic Flexation™ typically for between 2 and 3 seconds, or even for as long as 4 seconds if needed. This all takes place before beginning to count the required 7-second exercise time of the isometric contraction.

We prefer using one deep full breath in and out as a method of more accurately counting each second that has elapsed. This way, you will time each exercise more accurately, and you will not be tempted to hold your breath at any point which is a mistake that beginners often make.

Similarly, at the end of an exercise, we do not recommend that it be ended abruptly. Instead, we recommend reversing the Dynamic Flexation™ technique so that you gradually relax as you slightly move each muscle and joint out of the exercise position.

This process helps enormously because when you are in a good position it will help you to gain the maximum benefit from each exercise you perform. Dynamic Flexation™ is when you move and adjust either your feet, legs/leg, hips and especially your hands as you gradually assume a solid position and handgrip. As you flex and move, you will be making micro-adjustments.

All exercises will be performed best if you assume a correct and solid handgrip, fist clench, or foot position etc. One of the most important aspects of assuming the correct exercise position begins with your grip.

Without a solid grip on a bar, handle, or anything else you need to hold while exercising, you will naturally be setting yourself up to perform sub-maximally. You can also be helping to develop injuries which can include sore elbows, joints, ligaments, and tendons.

Dynamic Flexation™ is a concept that embraces the broader principles of motor unit recruitment, and "Henneman's Size Principle" to increase the contractile strength of a muscle. Elwood Henneman's principle stated that under load, the motor units in a muscle are engaged according to their magnitude of force output, from the smallest to the largest, and in task-appropriate order.

This means that the slow-twitch, low-force, fatigue-resistant muscle fibres are activated before any fast-twitch, high-force muscle fibres are engaged which are less fatigue-resistant. Since the body naturally works in this way, it enables precise and finely controlled force to be delivered at all levels of output.

This also means that when exercising, or when performing tasks in daily life, the fatigue which is experienced as a result will always be minimised. It will also be proportional to the sequential engagement of the most appropriate muscle fibres being engaged.

Isometric Exercises and Blood Pressure

Some exercise critics point out the fact that when someone performs an isometric exercise it will raise their blood pressure. However, the same people also very conveniently forget that the same is also true of all other forms of exercise including freehand callisthenics and traditional isotonic resistance training with weights.

ALL physical activity, and especially exercise will cause your blood pressure to rise for a short time. Providing that you are in good health you should always breathe deeply, naturally, and normally when performing any exercise, then any rise in blood pressure will soon return to a normal level when the exercise is stopped. The faster this happens, the fitter you are.

For those who are advanced athletes and/or are used to hard and intense isometric training for a long time, then you will already have made significant progress in strengthening your heart and circulatory system.

For those who are new to isometric training, just like with any form of exercise, the best way into it is by taking it slowly and less intensely at first.

Newcomers to exercise, and especially isometrics, should always focus on applying less intensity, to begin with, and on always breathing fully and deeply throughout all exercises. NEVER HOLD YOUR BREATH!

Under strict medical supervision, even those with Coronary Artery Disease and high blood pressure should be able to increase their physical activity levels with a reasonable degree of safety safely.

However, if you are a person who already suffers from high blood pressure, then you should always exercise at a much lower level of intensity than someone who has no physical issues.

Furthermore, **EVERYONE, AND ESPECIALLY PEOPLE WITH HYPERTENSION, OR ANY FORM OF CARDIOVASCULAR DISEASE, SHOULD ALWAYS CHECK WITH THEIR DOCTOR BEFORE BEGINNING ANY KIND OF EXERCISE ROUTINE.**

Rest and Recovery

When calculating your ideal recovery period, many things must be taken into consideration. These include your age, your current health and fitness level, the quantity of exercise taken, and most importantly the intensity of the exercise which has been performed.

Some people will need a recovery period of between 24 and 48 hours, and for others, the recovery period may be as brief as between 12 and 24 hours.

As a rule, the recovery period will always incrementally increase as the intensity of the exercises increases towards an individual's 100% potential maximum capacity. Always be aware of this and make sure that you factor this into your rest and recovery time calculations. The diagram will help to outline this.

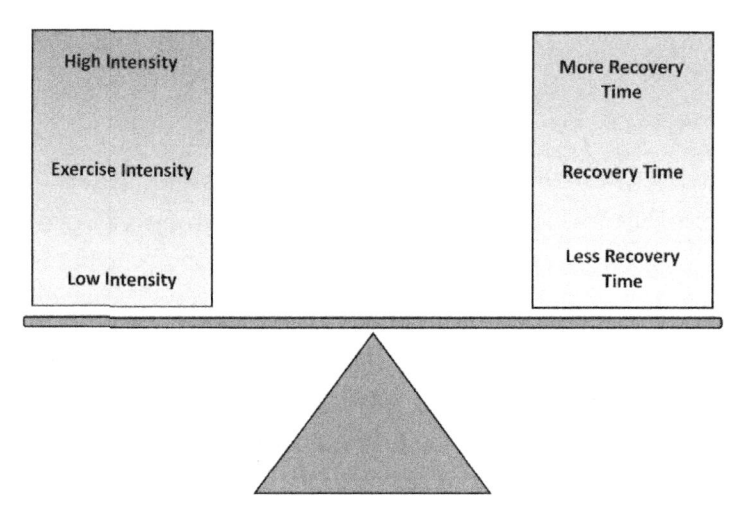

High Intensity		More Recovery Time
Exercise Intensity		Recovery Time
Low Intensity		Less Recovery Time

Sports scientist J. Atha's research revealed something remarkable. This was that when performing isometric contraction exercises at two-thirds of an individual's maximum capacity, the average person could safely perform an exercise like this daily, without overtraining.

Standard isometric contraction exercises can be safely performed daily, by almost anyone, of almost any age, and in almost any physical condition as a means of strength development, body shaping, and even bodybuilding.

However, for more intense workouts, then we recommend a full rest day between workouts due to the higher demands being placed upon the Central Nervous System (CNS) and the time needed to fully recover and benefit from the exercise.

Several other factors affect post-exercise recovery. These include a balanced and properly executed stretching routine and getting enough quality sleep. While you sleep, your body releases certain hormones which help you to repair and rebuild damaged tissue, and which will directly help your muscles to grow.

Adequate Nutrition is Vital

Quality post-exercise nutrition will help your body to repair itself faster, decrease your recovery time, and help to maximise the benefits gained from the exercise. Research shows that post-exercise immunodepression peaks if you exercise for longer than you are currently capable, and problems are enhanced due to reduced or inadequate nutrition. Hydration is also one of the most important factors in your recovery, as well as for your overall health, especially since your muscles are mostly composed of water.

Early studies suggested a 30 to 60-minute window after exercise when you need to eat, after which, your body begins to draw upon itself to repair and recover from your workout. Later studies found that this window can be anything from 1 to 3 hours depending on the workout type, intensity, and goals. On average, since most leave 60-minutes after food before hard exercise, and if a workout lasts an average of 45 minutes, then a 30 to 45-minute window to eat after exercise will mean it has been up to 150 minutes (2.5 hours) since your last food, therefore, the earlier suggested 30–45-minute window still makes sense for most people especially if they want to build more muscle and strength.

Most people mistakenly consume excessive amounts of protein at the expense of other key nutrients such as carbohydrates. Therefore, in doing this they are working against their best interests and overall optimum health. One of the key nutrients that have been found to help enormously when in recovery from prolonged periods of heavy exercise is carbohydrates. A lot of research supports the hypothesis that carbohydrate is the most important nutritional factor in preventing post-exercise immunodepression. Most do not realise that the protein composition of human muscle is typically only somewhere in the region of between 18/9% and 21% protein (average 20%) and the rest is made up of water, glucose, lipids, and carbohydrates etc. We will not go into more detail here, however, if you want to learn more about this and many other surprising nuggets of useful information about sensible nutrition and exercise then they can be found in The 70 Second Difference book.

Strength, Stamina, Endurance, and Resilience

It is important to understand the difference between strength, stamina and endurance because once understood, you will then be able to devise the most suitable workout routines according to your body type.

Muscular strength is possibly best understood as being a muscle's capacity to exert force against resistance, or weight. This is comparatively easy to measure because your ability to lift a given amount of weight for a single repetition is a good measure of your strength.

Stamina is the length of time at which a muscle, or group of muscles, can perform at or near its maximum capacity. For example, the number of squats you can perform with a given weight which is 90% of your maximum would be a measure of your stamina or the distance which you can carry a similarly heavy object such as an anvil.

Endurance is all about time, and your ability to perform a certain muscular action for a prolonged period regardless of the capacity at which you are working.

Resilience is all about your ability to recover from whatever stresses and demands are placed on your muscles. However, resilience is mostly all about your state of mind, your mental toughness and ability to endure, perform and deliver under pressure, and how you recover quickly emotionally.

The muscular composition of your body will always determine how well you will perform in certain sports. The amount of slow twitch muscle fibres you possess will determine how well you perform at endurance-related events, and both type A and type B fast twitch muscle fibres are all about explosive power and your ability to maintain it.

In simple terms, if you possess mostly slow twitch fibres, then you are naturally going to be better suited to endurance sports. Alternatively, if you possess mostly fast twitch muscle fibres, then you are a natural weightlifter. It is important to note, that no matter what your natural predisposition might be in this respect, with the correct training regimen, it is still possible to significantly increase your abilities in your naturally weaker opposing areas of speciality.

Chapter 3: Improvised and Proprietary Isometric Exercise Equipment

One of the best things about isometric exercises is that if you do not want to use traditional gym equipment or proprietary devices, then you do not have to use them to perform a full workout. Instead, you can either use nothing at all except your own body, immovable objects such as doors, walls, and door jambs, or readily available everyday items. These can include walking sticks/poles, broom handles, towels and sturdy towing, or a climbing rope. I will lay out some of these items as suggestions for alternative equipment/devices you can use for your workout sessions.

Improvised Isometric Exercise Devices
Rope – Either Climbing Rope or Towing Rope

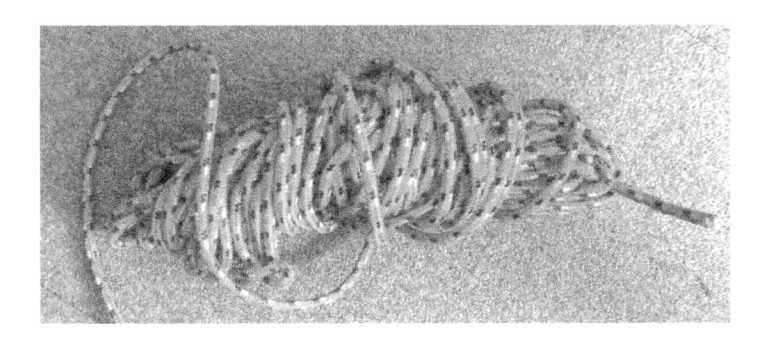

A rope is another simple but highly effective tool that can be used to perform an isometric and/or self-resisted workout routine. the important things to look for in a rope that might be suitable for exercise use are, sufficient length, it must be thick enough to allow a comfortable handgrip, and it must be in good condition so that it will not break during your workout routine.

If you are using your feet to secure the rope, then for added safety and comfort you may wish to loop the rope around the foot as shown. This will make it less likely to slip when it is pulled hard, and it will be more comfortable for the foot as well.

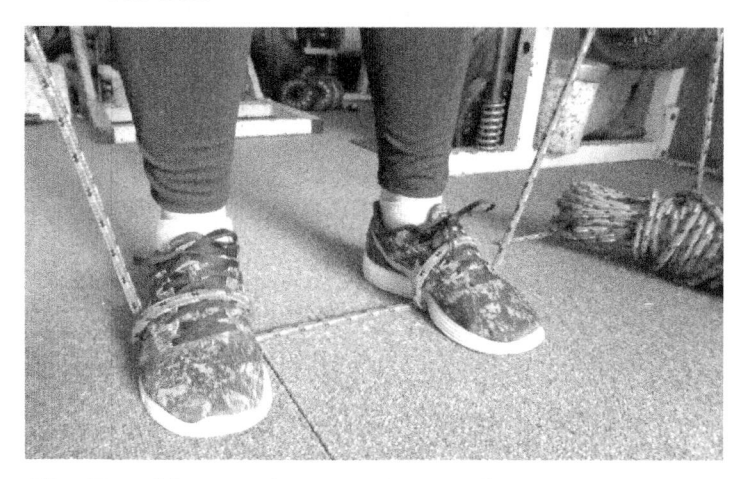

The Humble Beach or Bath Towel

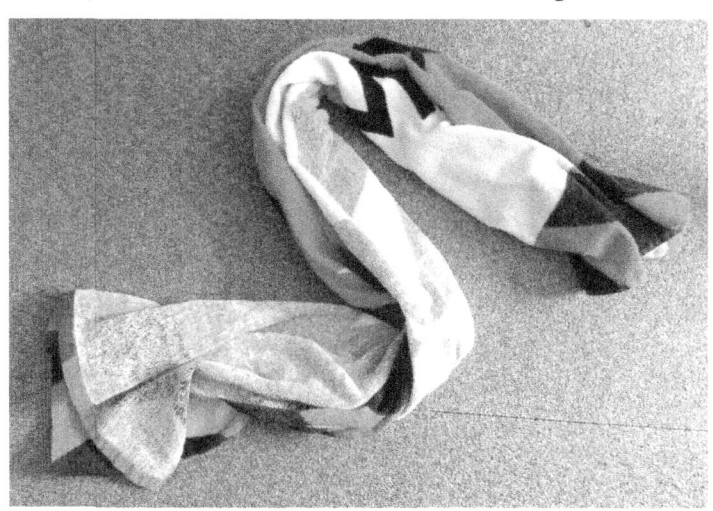

The humble beach or bath towel is a common tool used by isometric enthusiasts who have nothing else to exercise with. It is also an exercise tool of choice for many because it is incredibly versatile. When choosing a towel to exercise with, the important things to look for are that it must be long enough, it must also be flexible enough to enable you to grip it properly, and therefore, it must not be too thick. Naturally, it must also be in good condition and not be liable to tear or rip during your exercise session.

The Broom Handle

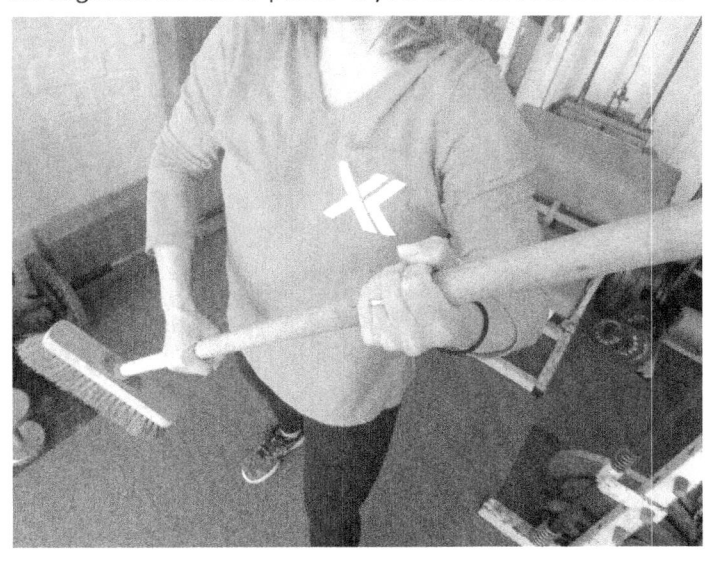

The broom handle can be used almost identically to the walking stick or pro-style walking pole. By its very nature, it is not nearly as flexible as a walking stick or pro-style walking pole. This is because you can easily take a walking stick or pro-style walking pole virtually anywhere because that is precisely what they have been designed for. You would appear to be very odd indeed if you were to carry around a broom with you to exercise with, whereas a walking stick or pro-style walking pole would not look even the slightest bit out of place. If you use a broom handle at home to exercise with, then make sure it is solid and will not break when used in a workout routine. Also, we would strongly caution against using one to support your body weight in any way with the broom handle to support it.

The Walking Stick/Pole

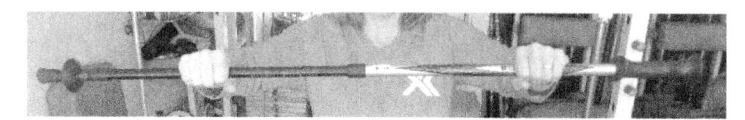

The walking stick or pro-style walking pole is an excellent device to use for an isometric workout. It is an improvised equivalent of a barbell or Bullworker® Classic without the steel cables at each side. One of the great advantages the pro-style walking pole offers is that it can be adjusted to various lengths, which makes it easily adaptable for use in a variety of exercises.

Many of the exercises can be performed alone, without any need for partner assistance. An even greater range of exercises can be performed if a workout partner is available. Nordic Walking Poles are different from ordinary walking poles, but they work equally well for isometric exercises.

Photo: Daniel Case

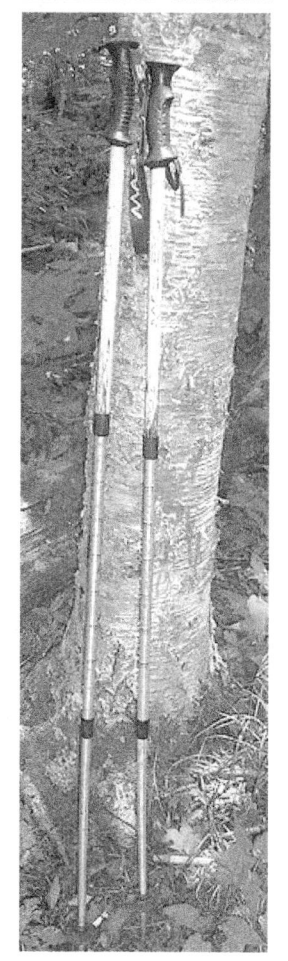

Proprietary Isometric Exercise Equipment

We highly recommend and endorse the Iso-Bow® as an excellent exercise tool. This inexpensive little device is an amazingly versatile device that allows self-resisted isometric exercises to be performed very easily. It also allows self-resisted isotonic and what I call functional isokinetic exercises to be performed easily too. The Iso-Bow® provides the user with a biomechanically sound grip handle which allows almost all exercises to be performed more effectively, and with greater ease and comfort.

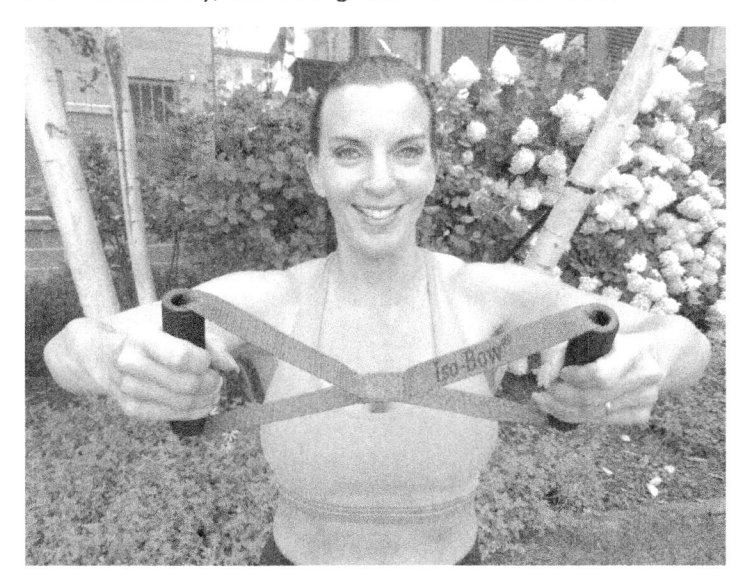

With a pair of Iso-Bows®, you can effectively exercise every major muscle group of the body, and even perform advanced exercises such as the pull-up, the squat, and the deadlift. The level of workout you can get from using a pair of Iso-Bows® can range from an easy low-level beginner's workout, right up to a very high-intensity professional athlete level of workout. Amazingly, you can do all of this without any adjustment being needed to the Iso-Bows®. Each user will benefit proportionately, according to the amount of effort and intensity that is applied during each exercise.

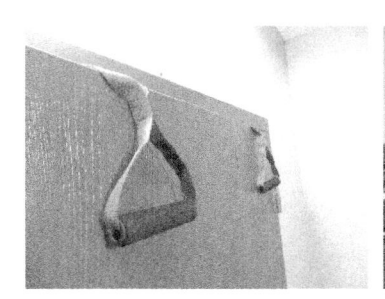

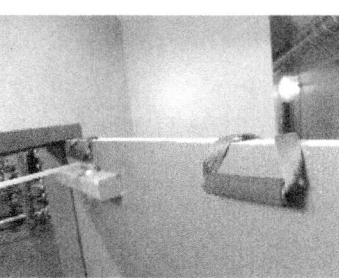

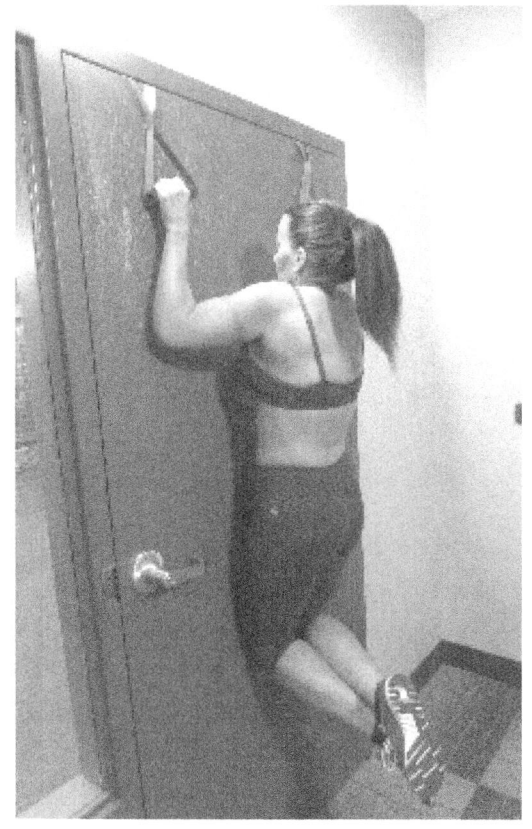

Even a pair of Iso-Bows® are so compact they can easily fit into the average jacket or jeans pocket, a small handbag/purse, a briefcase, or a walking rucksack or bag.

Perhaps the best-known of all isometric/isotonic home exercise devices is the Bullworker® which has been a best-seller since it was launched in the early 1960s. Today, it is still a best-selling device, and with good reason, because it works. The smaller "partner" device is called the Steel Bow®, and both have interchangeable springs so that both men and women of all strength levels and abilities can use them, with roughly equal effectiveness.

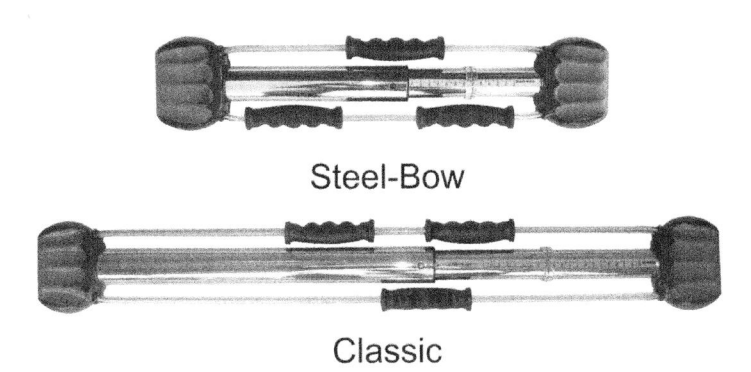

Steel-Bow

Classic

Securing the Iso-Bow® With Your Feet

When performing leg exercises such as squats, split squats, and lunges, as well as lower back and glute exercises such as the deadlift, it becomes necessary to properly secure the Iso-Bow® using your feet. There are several ways in which the Iso-Bow® can be secured using your feet, and your personal preference of how you do this will depend upon many factors such as your foot size, your choice of footwear, and ease of operation.

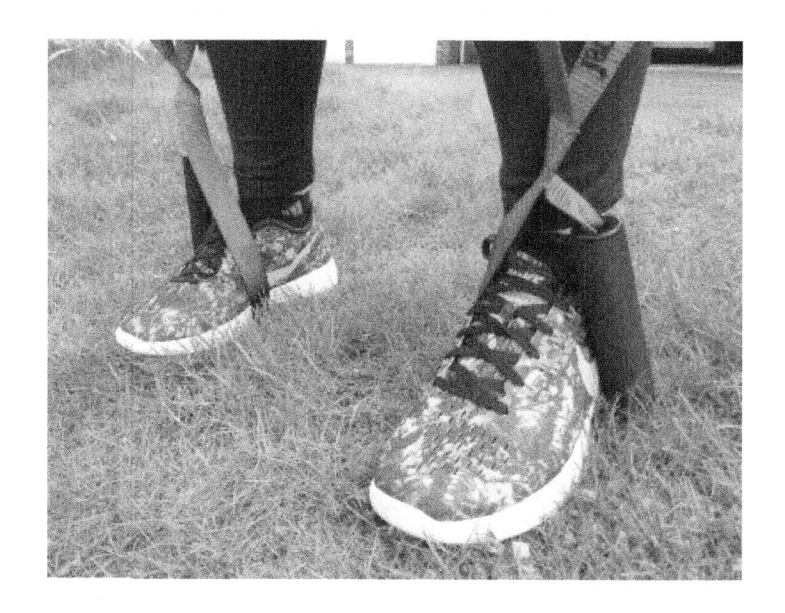

You can secure the Iso-Bow® with your foot inside one of the handles. You do this by adjusting the handgrip to one side, usually the outer side of the foot, and then placing your feet inside the loop like a stirrup.

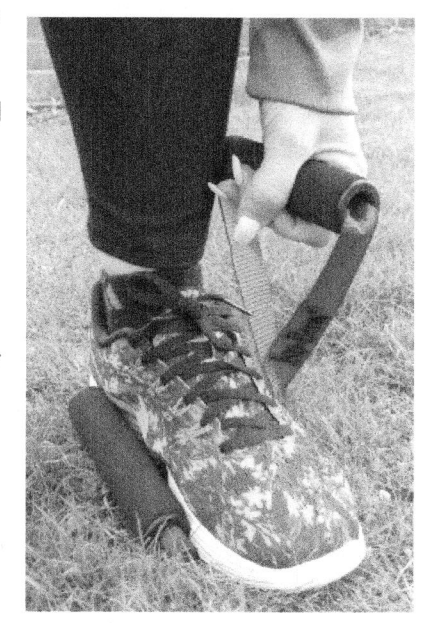

Another method is to place the Iso-Bow® flat on the floor and then stand on one side of the straps so that the handle of the same side sits flush with your inner foot. In this position, it will be your bodyweight combined with the handle pressing against the inner side of your foot which enables you to pull safely and securely.

The final method is to simply place each foot through one end of an Iso-Bow®, stepping onto the foam hand grip as you do so. This method is slightly less stable than the other two methods.

However, if the foot can be pushed far enough through the loop of the Iso-Bow® handle, then the handle will slightly raise the level of your heel making it easier for some people to squat.

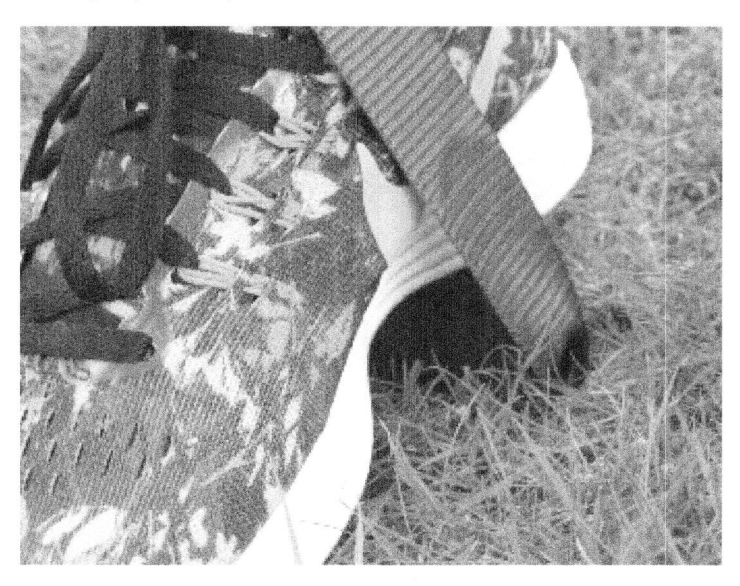

Naturally, safety is always a top priority so whichever method you ultimately choose to use, you should always make sure that when securing the Iso-Bow® with your feet that there is never any chance of it slipping in any way while you exercise.

Chapter 4: Direct Comparisons

The pictures In this section show a direct comparison between a selection of martial arts moves, techniques and stances and an isometric exercise that relates to them. This is to demonstrate how the performance of a certain isometric exercise can directly improve the performance of the moves and techniques being demonstrated. It is not a great leap of vision to imagine how strength conditioning in this way will help to improve your performance in all aspects of your martial art.

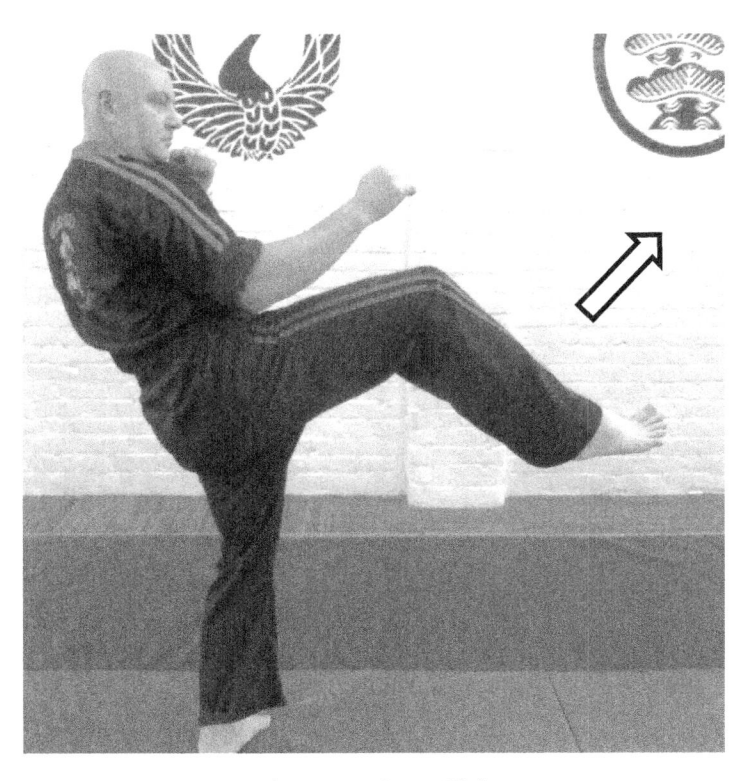

Comparison 1

The Front Snap Kick

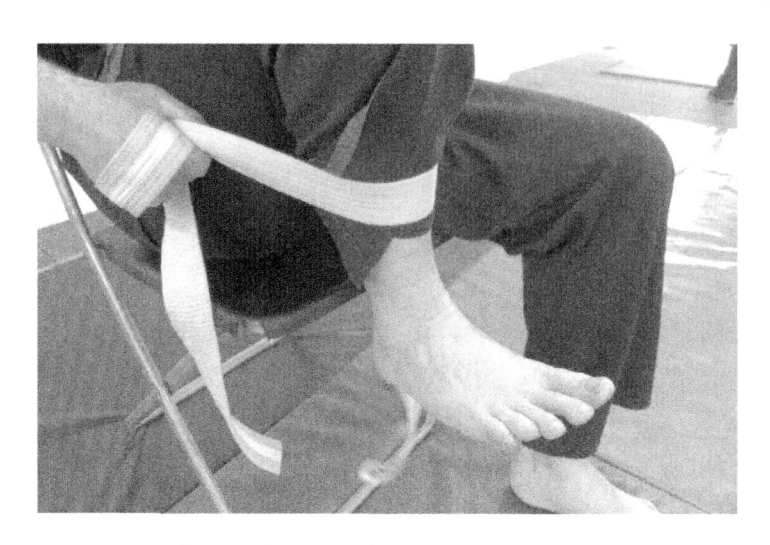

The Single Leg Belt Extension Exercise

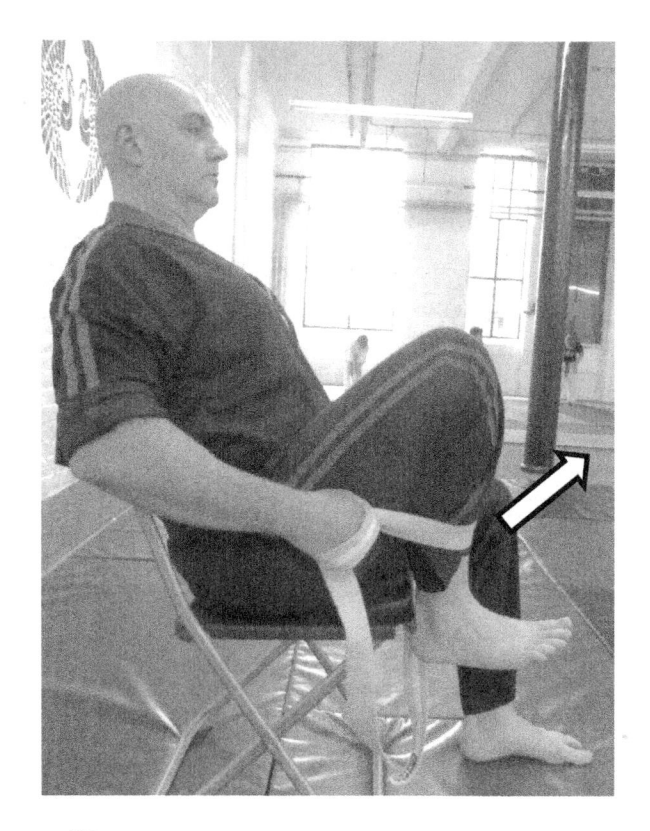

Comparison 2

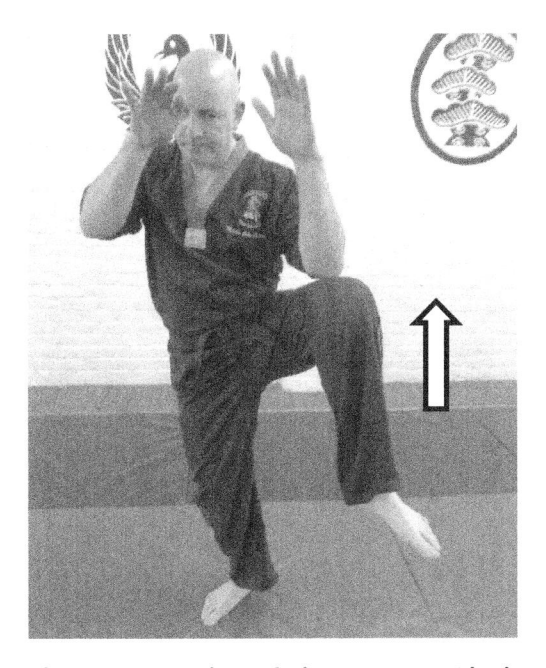

The Knee Attack, and The Knee-Leg Block

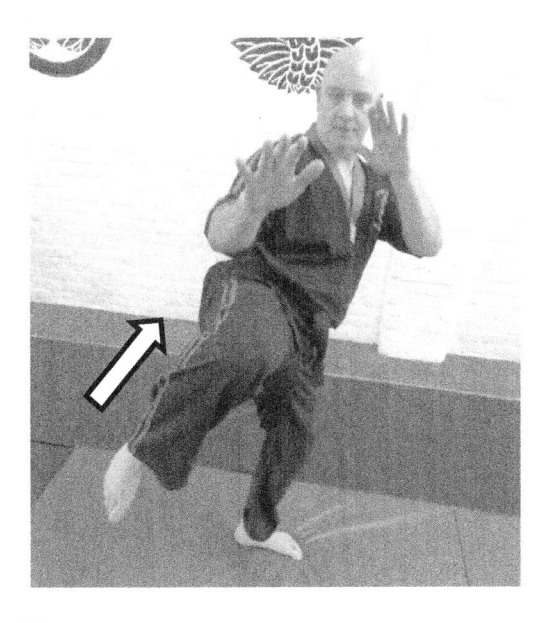

The Single Leg Belt Extension Exercise

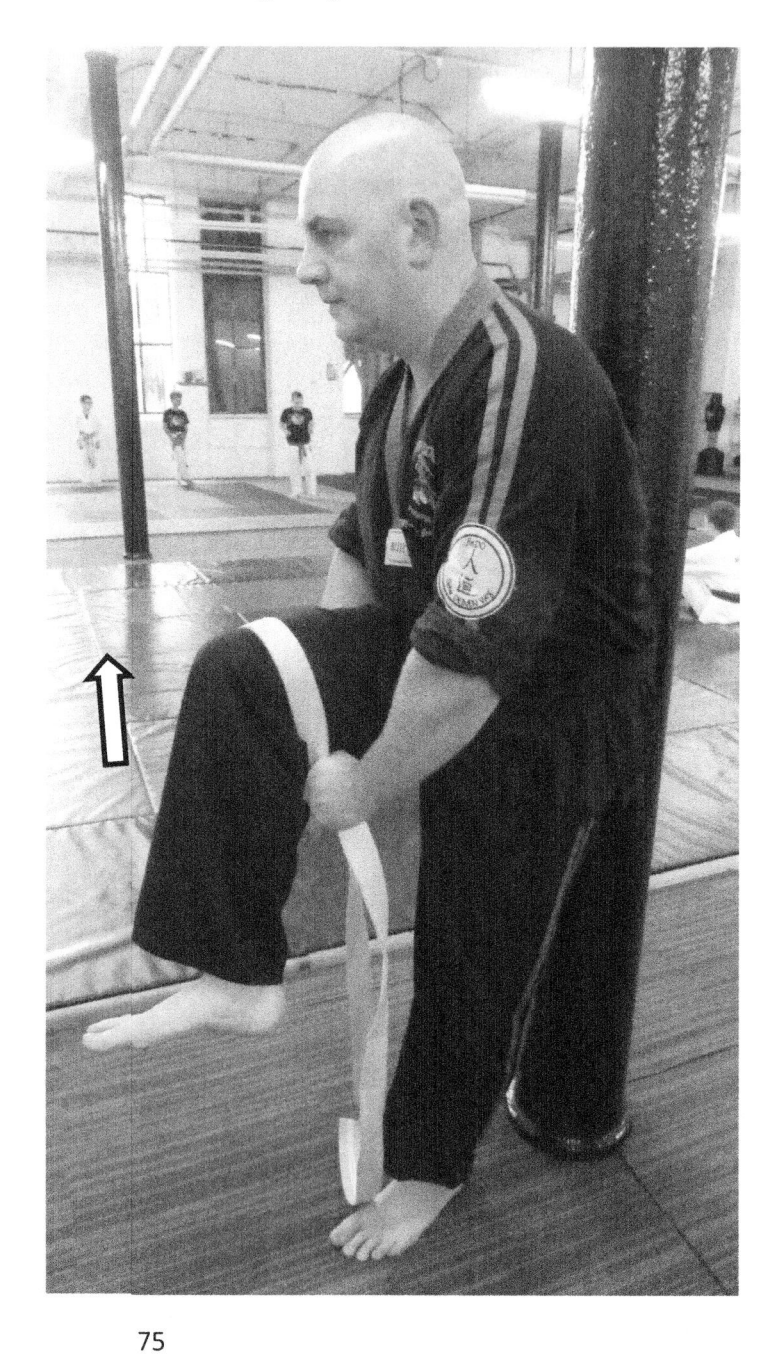

Comparison 3

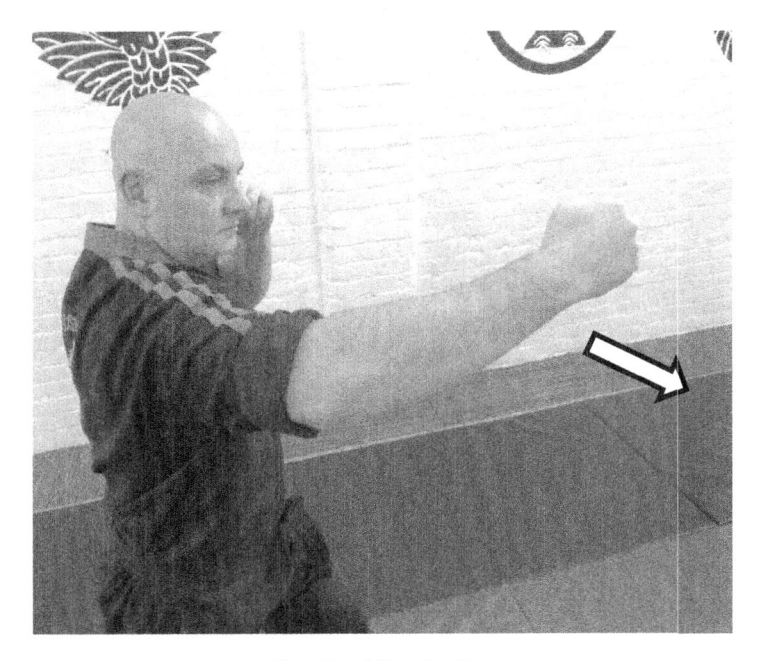

The Backfist Strike

Triceps Side Extension Backfist Exercise

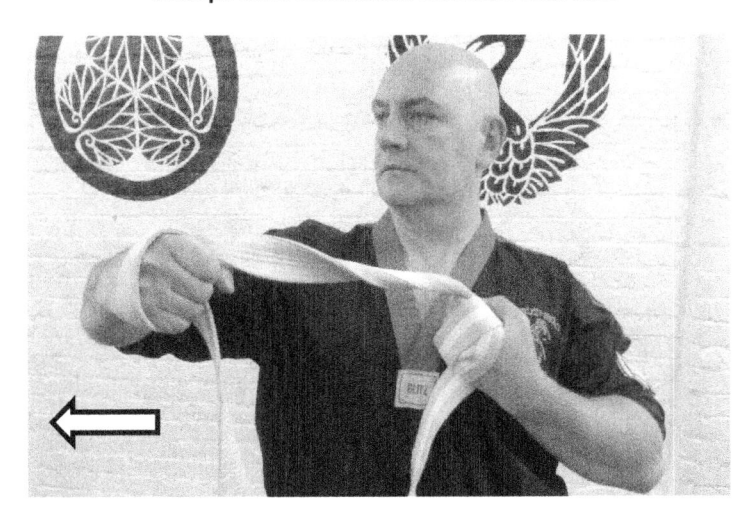

Comparison 4

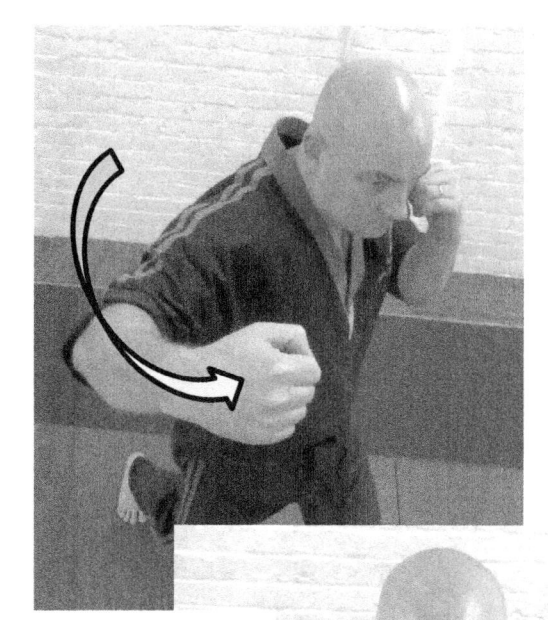

The Hook Punch

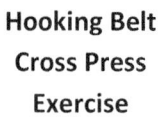

Hooking Belt Cross Press Exercise

77

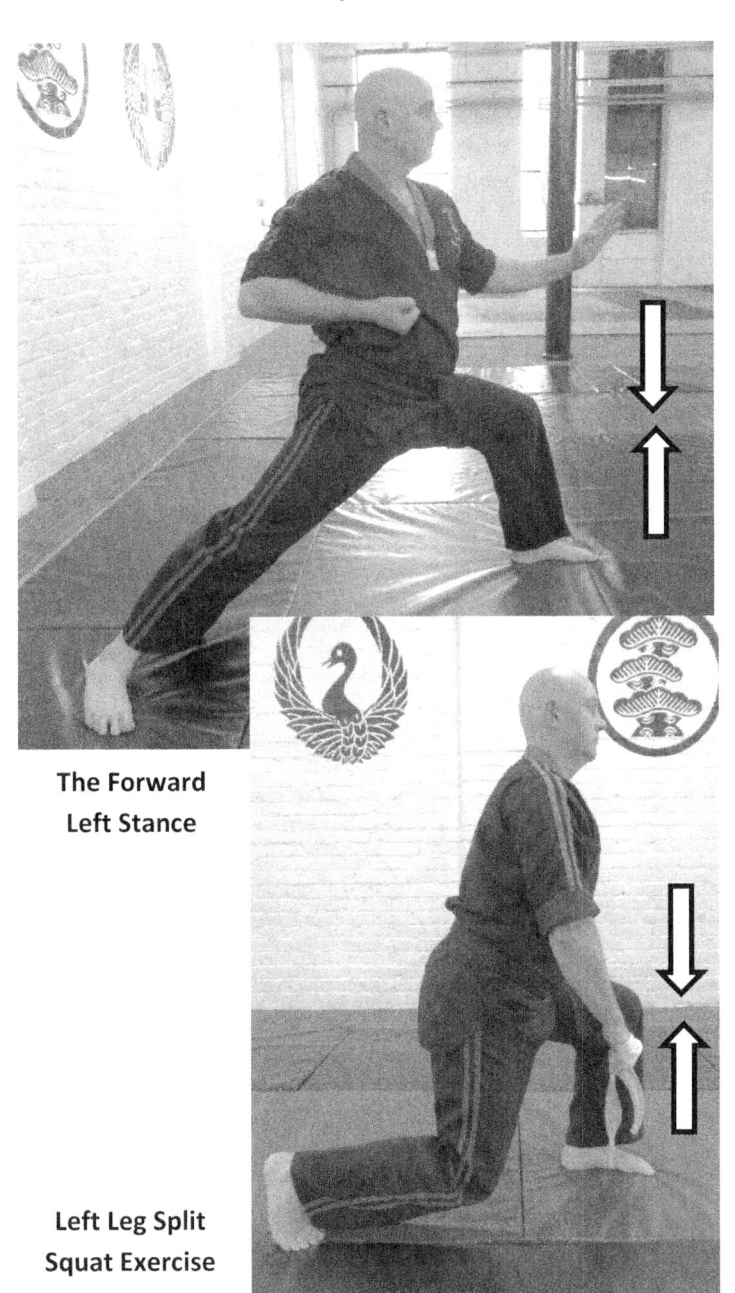

Comparison 5

The Forward Left Stance

Left Leg Split Squat Exercise

These few examples of how a specific martial arts strike, stance or block etc. can be improved directly through performing an isometric exercise that follows the same or similar biomechanical action. It is worth taking the time to think about this and to consider just how many more exercises you can perform that will directly improve your performance in a specific way. It does not matter which martial art you practice because there will always be an equivalent isometric exercise performance enhancer that can be practised as part of your conditioning programme.

Chapter 5:
Things to Remember Before You Begin

- The first and perhaps the most important thing to remember is: **NEVER HOLD YOUR BREATH AT ANY TIME.**
- Breathing in and out naturally during all isometric exercises will also help you count the number of elapsed seconds much more accurately, with one full breath in and out taking approximately one second.
- We recommend that you read the instructions about each exercise carefully. You can also watch the associated videos via the TWiEA™ website if you wish to become a member and access the resource.
- Always leave a safe distance between you and others if exercising with any proprietary device or IIED (Improvised Isometric Exercise Device)
- Always check the structural integrity of any type of exercise device. If there is any doubt about the structural integrity, then do not use it for exercise or any other purpose.
- Double-check that any/all adjustable joints on the exercise device and/or IIED are secure before use.
- Weight loss/fat loss will ONLY occur when any exercise plan is used in conjunction with a calorie-controlled diet.
- It is critically important to completely focus your mind on the exercise being performed. Envision the muscle you are exercising as growing larger and stronger.

⚠ Always consult a professional coach to devise a detailed stretching routine, this will ensure that you are stretching the areas effectively rather than risking injury.

⚠ Always ensure that a stable line of biomechanical progression is achieved before engaging in and performing any exercise.

⚠ Warming-up, stretching, and cooling down are three of the most overlooked yet essential elements to exercise, and we cannot stress their importance strongly enough.

⚠ During ANY form of physical exercise, including isometrics, if you apply too much intensity too soon, then you may inadvertently strain a muscle. Isometric exercise is particularly intense, and a single isometric exercise engages a great many more muscle fibres than even high-intensity weight training, and isometrics engages the muscle fibres at a much higher level too.

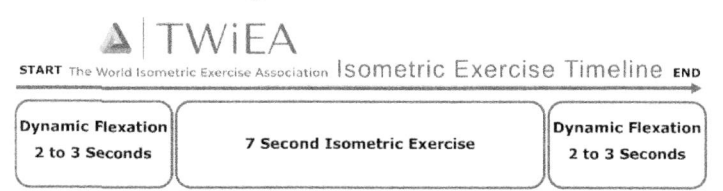

⚠ | TWiEA

START The World Isometric Exercise Association Isometric Exercise Timeline END

| Dynamic Flexation | 7 Second Isometric Exercise | Dynamic Flexation |
| 2 to 3 Seconds | | 2 to 3 Seconds |

For safety's sake, we always recommend using Dynamic Flexation™ to engage your muscles gradually and progressively into ANY exercise, especially isometrics, according to what we call The ISOfitness Exercise Engagement Timeline™.

The main benefit of properly warming up for several minutes before a workout is injury prevention and increasing your heart rate and circulation to your muscles, ligaments, and tendons. It is important to remember that warming-up and stretching are two different concepts and that stretching is not a good warm-up. This is because stretching will put the muscle in an un-contracted position and weaken it. Stretching is always best performed after a workout has been completed, together with a proper cool-down. In addition to properly warming-up, always perform a gentle flex and stretch of the muscles and joints which are about to be exercised. For example, squatting down fully to flex the thighs and loosen the knees is always a good idea before performing any leg exercises. Dynamic Flexation™ performed before any exercise should help to ensure greater great flexibility and increased blood supply to the muscles and surrounding tissue.

Isometric exercises are deceptively powerful. Even when engaging in what may feel like only moderate-intensity exercise, you are probably still engaging and contracting many more muscle fibres than you would in a similar isotonic exercise. Therefore, if you are in any doubt whatsoever, then always perform the exercise with a little less intensity.

All exercises and workout plans work equally well for men and women. Both sexes can build strength, muscle, body build, or simply get into great shape if so desired, each according to their natural ability.

In our exercise resource books, the exercises listed are suggestions of what can be performed for each body part/muscle group. We are not suggesting that they should all be performed. Instead, users may wish to select the most suitable exercises from each section. In our course books, please perform the exercises according to the workout session notes.

Finally, please read, review, and ensure that you have fully complied with all recommendations in the section entitled: 'Important General Safety and Health Guidelines,' and only start using the isometric, or any exercise system with the full approval of your physician.

Equipment

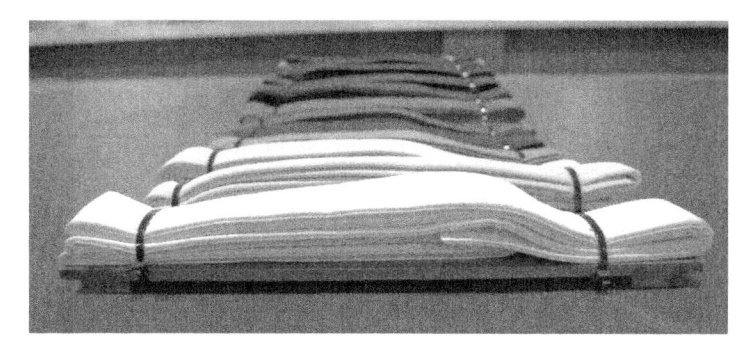

The standard martial arts belt is a strong item made from cotton webbing (or similar) construction. In East Asian martial arts, the belt colour is associated with the level of expertise of the wearer. The systematic use of belt colour to denote rank was first used in Japan by Jigoro Kano, the founder of judo in the 1880s. Today, these belts, or similar, are commonplace in most martial arts studios. Furthermore, they are easy and inexpensive to purchase if one is needed specifically for isometric exercise purposes.

An excellent alternative to using a martial arts belt would be a length of strong climbing rope. However, this does have the drawback of not being flat when placed under the feet during certain exercises such as the squat, and deadlift. This is also true during the overhead press where it may need to be placed under the knees if it is not long enough to be used under the feet. As an alternative to both the standard martial arts belt and climbing rope, strong shipping webbing (or similar) webbing can be used. In particular, the type of webbing is often used to construct commercial and domestic lifting straps.

A pair of plastic bottles with screw tops are an excellent resource to use in exercising grip strength. Make sure that the bottles are full to the brim with still water, and never use bottles containing a carbonated liquid in case it causes the bottles to burst during a sudden expansion. Additional pairs of bottles of different sizes are also useful tools because they vary the size of the handgrip which allows multiple exercise positions to be performed.

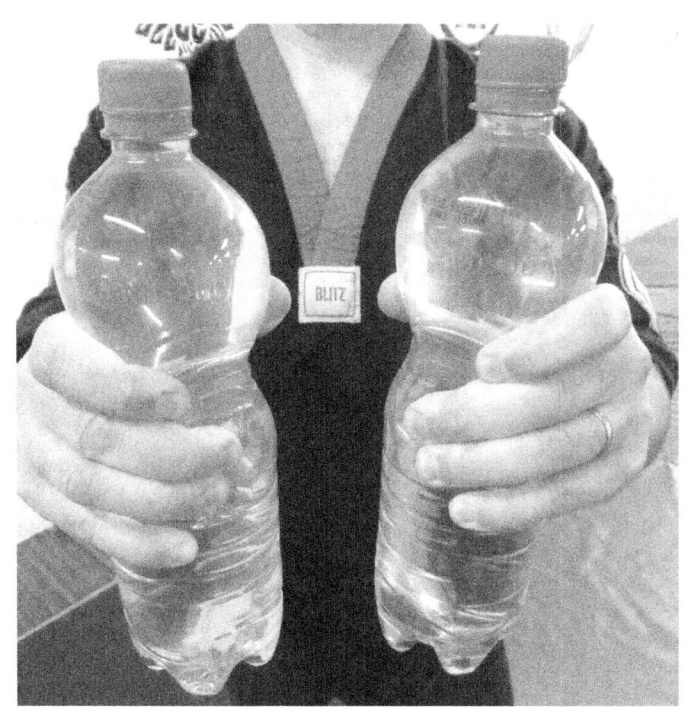

Chapter 6: About the Exercise Models

With special thanks to Sensei Marc Knowles who is a Chief Kickboxing Instructor, 1st Dan Freestyle Karate, 4th Dan: Kickboxing, a Reiki Master, and Senior Bushido Martial Arts Instructor. TWiEA™ (The World Isometric Exercise Association Accredited) Isometric Exercise Instructor.

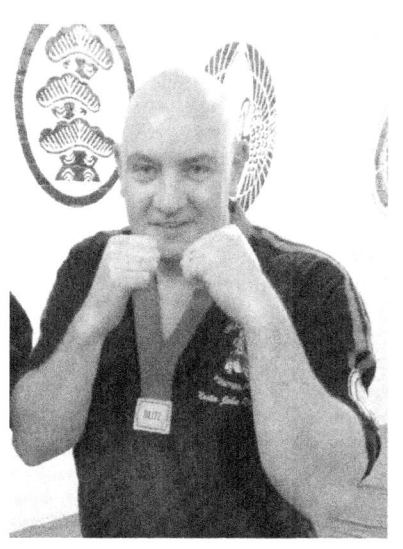

Contact: https://www.linkedin.com/company/synergy-performance-fitness-ltd/ - and/or www.TWiEA.com - and/or https://www.facebook.com/getsynergyfit

With special thanks to Senior Instructor Sensei Jacob Haynes, 2nd Dan Jiu-Jitsu WKC 10 times World Champion 2015 -2017, 1st Dan Freestyle Karate Traditional, Weapons & Creative Weapons, Jiu-Jitsu & Freestyle Karate English, and European Multi Kata Champion.

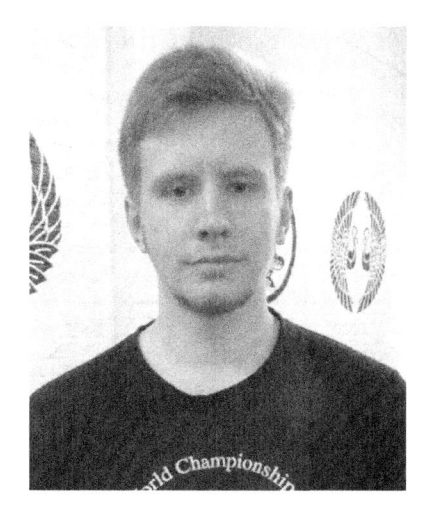

I would like to extend my special thanks to Bushido Martial Arts Chief Instructor Master John D. Robertson, 7th Dan: Shotokan Karate, 7th Dan: Freestyle Karate, 7th Dan: Jiu-Jitsu, WKC England Kata Team Manager, WKC World President Kata & Forms, WKC World Kickboxing / Points Fighting Referee.

Photoshoot Location

Bushido Martial Arts, Welkin Mill, Welkin Road, Stockport, SK6 2BH, England - www.bushidoma.co.uk

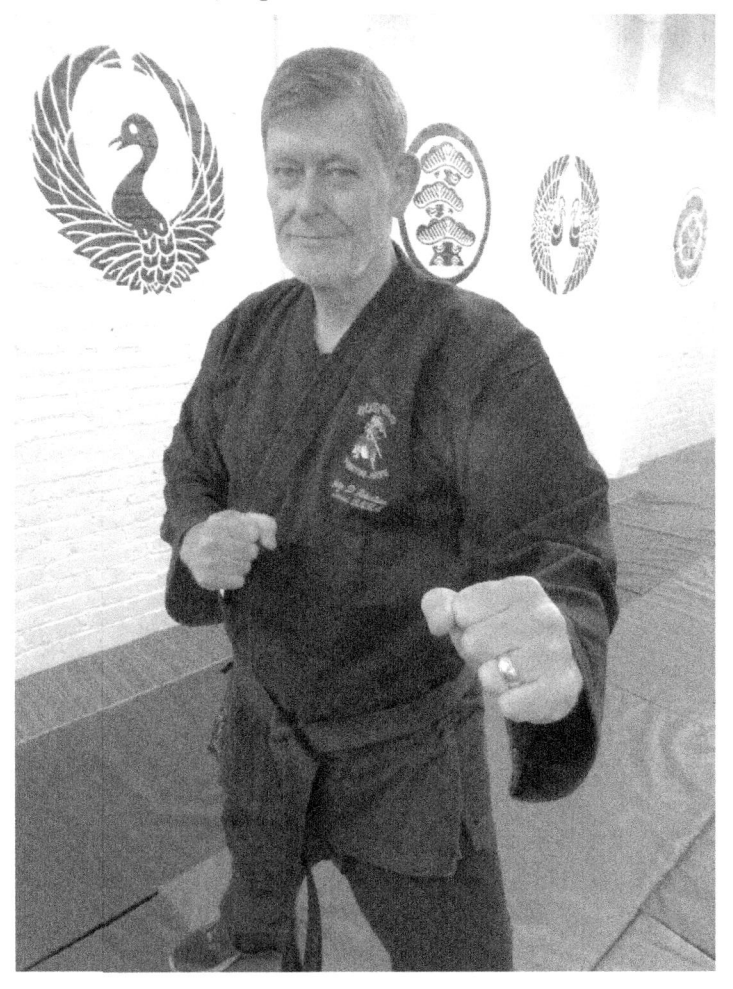

Chapter 7: Exercise Resources
Abdominals - Floor Stomach Crunch-Push

Lay with your back on the floor, with your knees bent and with your feet flat on the floor. Curl the torso upwards into the abdominal crunch position. This is not any sort of traditional sit-up. Instead, it is similar to imagining curling your upper body around a large imaginary ball. Either halfway through or towards the upper part of the curl, hold the position and then push back with your hands on your upper thighs. This will provide as much resistance as you need to perform the isometric exercise.

The harder you engage the muscles, the more intense the exercise becomes, so always be sure to exercise at an intensity that best suits your current ability. When you perform an isometric exercise never hold your breath.

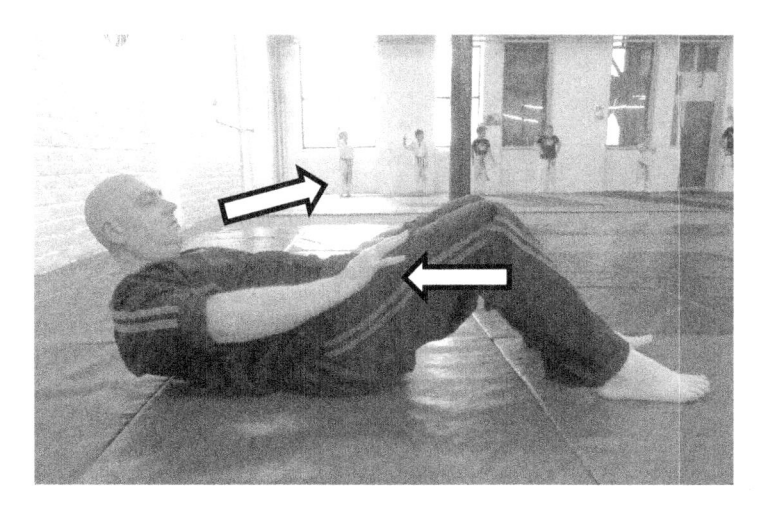

Always breathe deeply and naturally, which will be about 10 full breaths in and out at a rate of about 1 second per full breath. Perform each exercise for no less than 7 seconds, and no longer than 10.

89

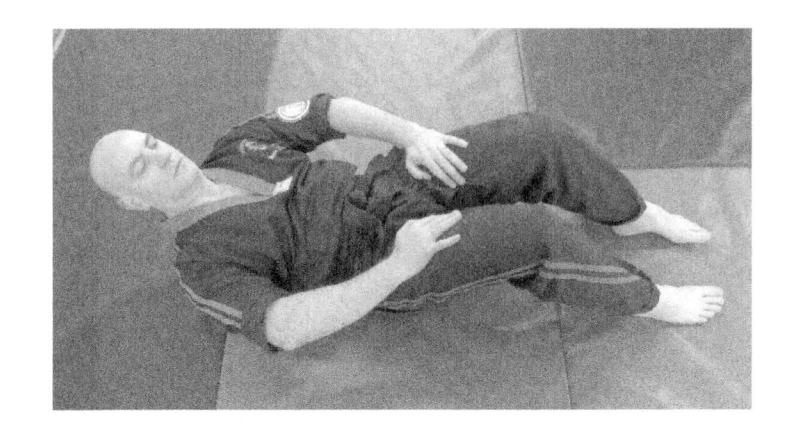

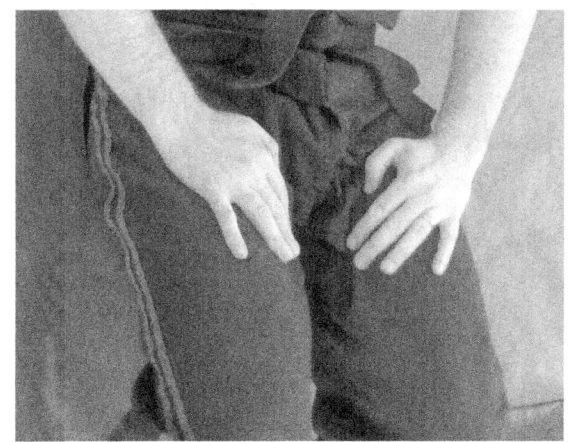

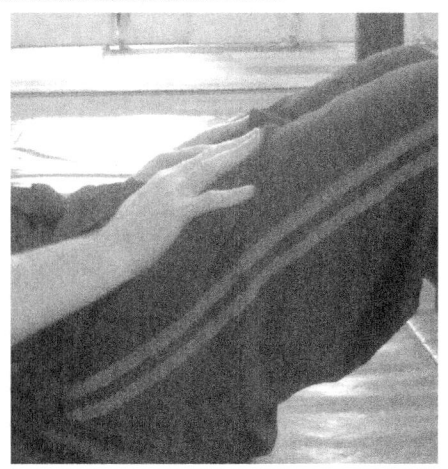

Abdominals – Seated Knee Raise Trunk Curl

Sit upright on a chair, bench, or any solid object. Take an ordinary martial arts belt, or similar, in both hands and place it over the top of one knee.

As you simultaneously raise the knee and leg slightly, push down on the knee using your stomach muscles as the driving force in a crunch-like movement.

Keep your elbows slightly bent and arms locked in that position throughout. As you push back with your hands on your knee/thighs it will provide as much resistance as you need to perform the isometric exercise.

This exercise can be performed with or without a martial arts belt. If no belt is used, then simply place the hands over the top of the knee/thigh and perform the rest of the exercise in the same way. Be sure to exercise both sides of the body by changing legs/knees etc.

The harder you engage the muscles, the more intense the exercise becomes, so always be sure to exercise at an intensity that best suits your current ability. When you perform an isometric exercise never hold your breath.

Always breathe deeply and naturally, which will be about 10 full breaths in and out at a rate of about 1 second per full breath. Perform each exercise for no less than 7 seconds, and no longer than 10.

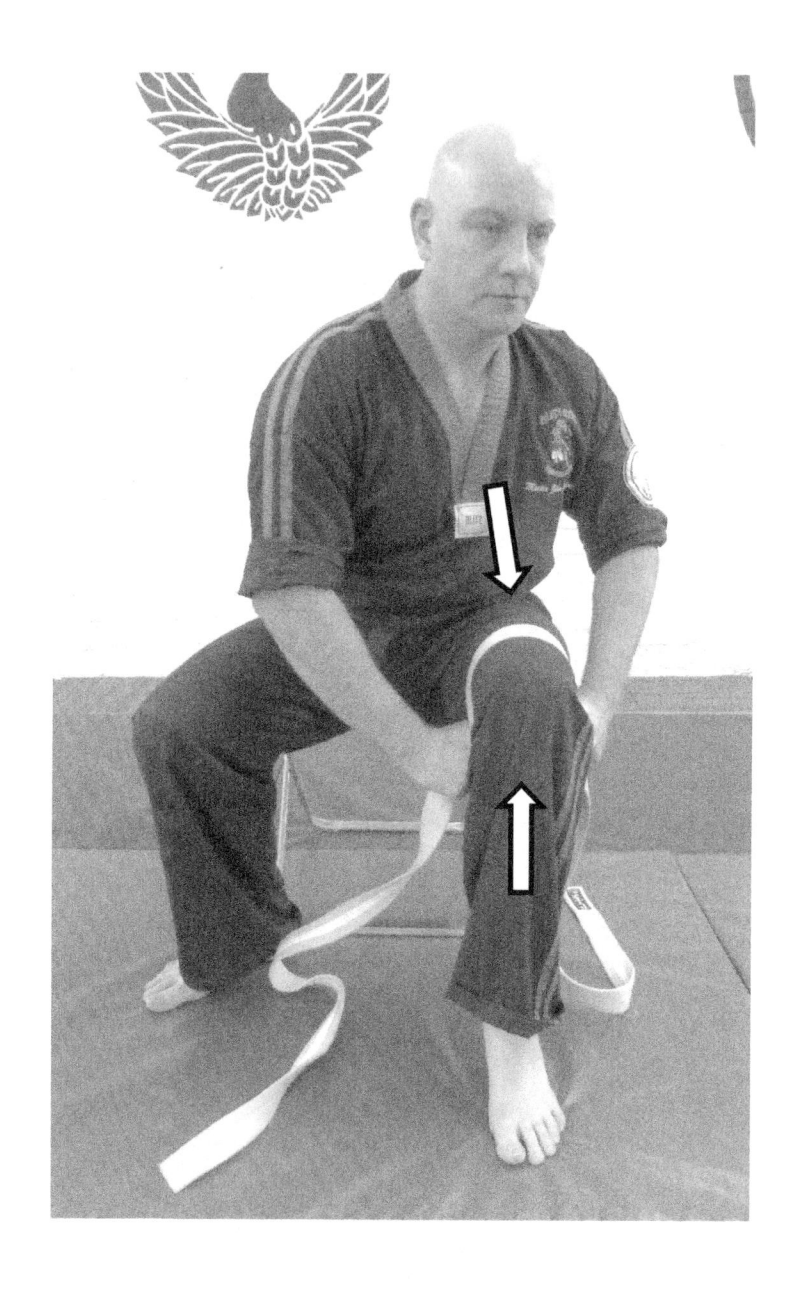

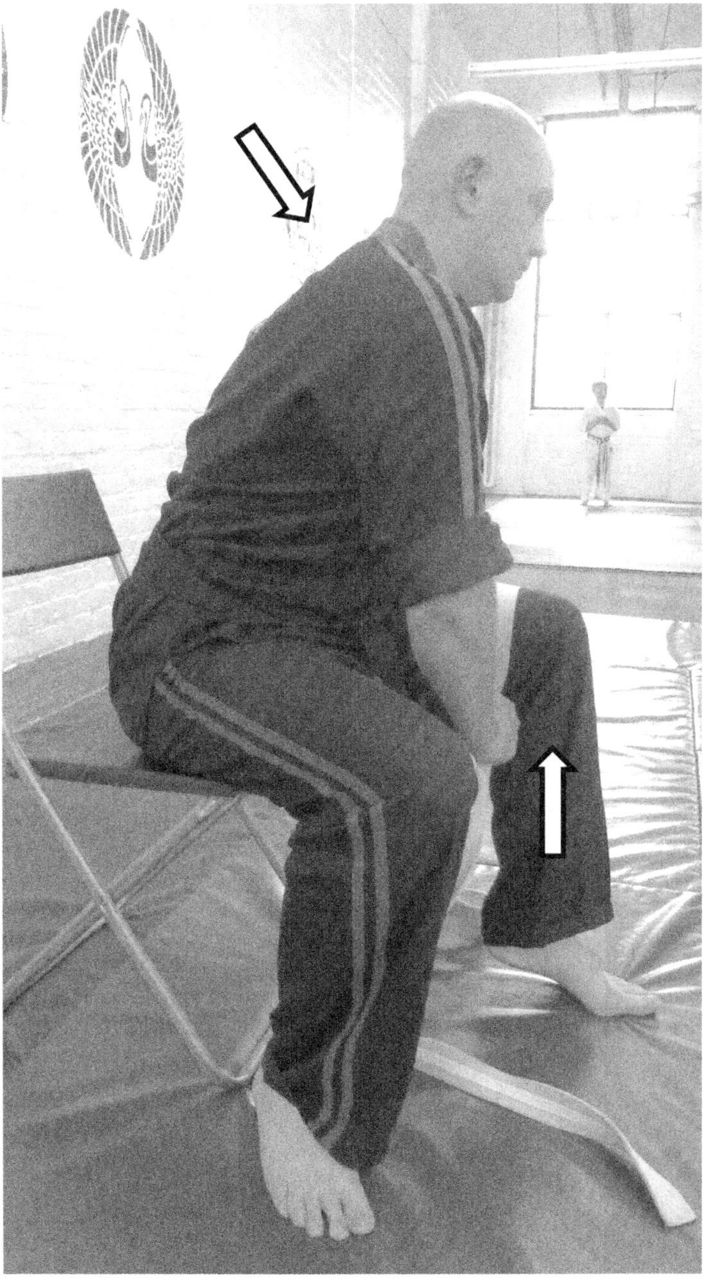

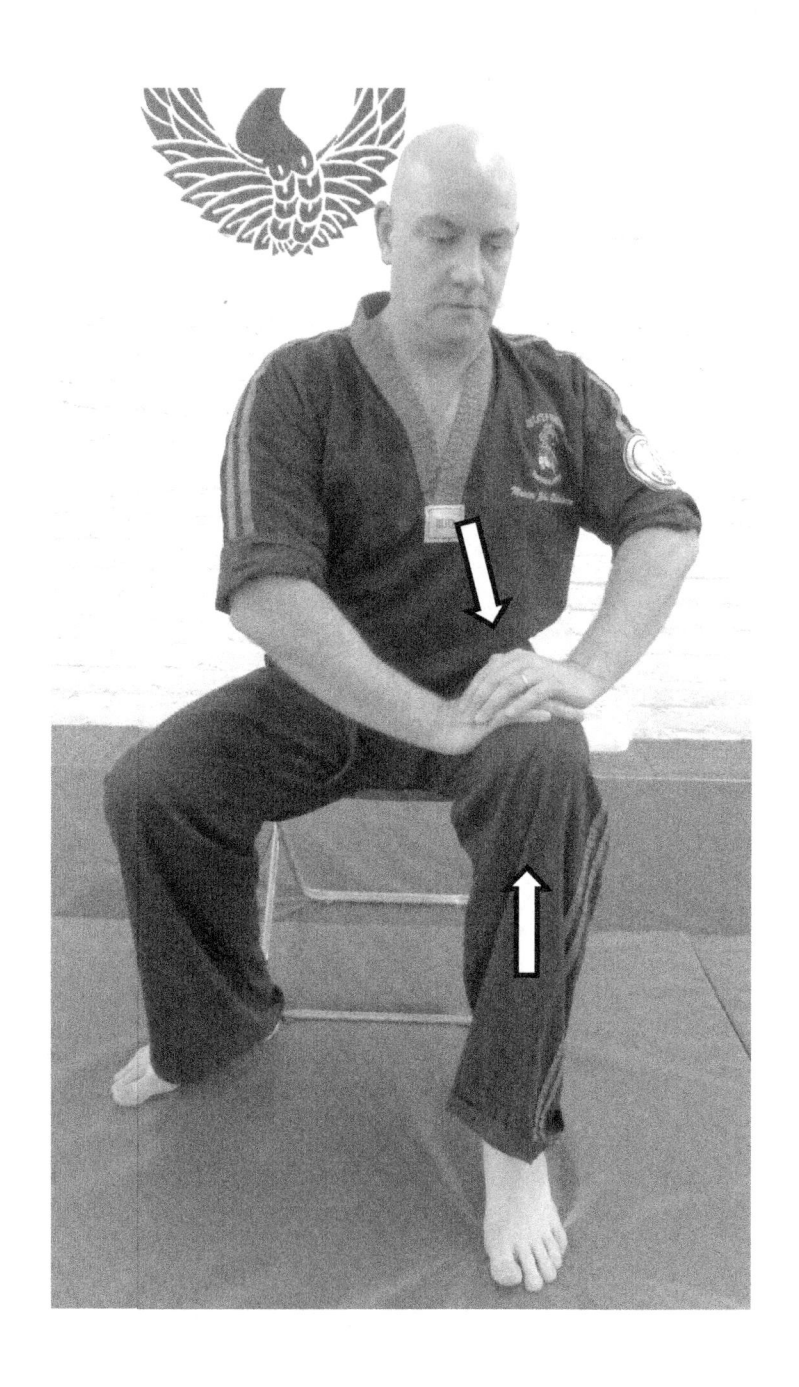

Abdominals – Standing Knee Raise Trunk Curl

Stand upright and lean back against a wall or any other solid object. Raise one leg/knee. Take an ordinary martial arts belt, or similar, in both hands and place it over the top of the knee.

As you simultaneously raise the knee and leg slightly, push down on the knee using your stomach muscles as the driving force in a crunch-like movement.

Keep your elbows slightly bent and arms locked in that position throughout. As you push back with your hands on your knee/thighs it will provide as much resistance as you need to perform the isometric exercise.

This exercise can be performed with or without a martial arts belt. If no belt is used, then simply place the hands over the top of the knee/thigh and perform the rest of the exercise in the same way. Be sure to exercise both sides of the body by changing legs/knees etc.

The harder you engage the muscles, the more intense the exercise becomes, so always be sure to exercise at an intensity that best suits your current ability. When you perform an isometric exercise never hold your breath.

Always breathe deeply and naturally, which will be about 10 full breaths in and out at a rate of about 1 second per full breath. Perform each exercise for no less than 7 seconds, and no longer than 10.

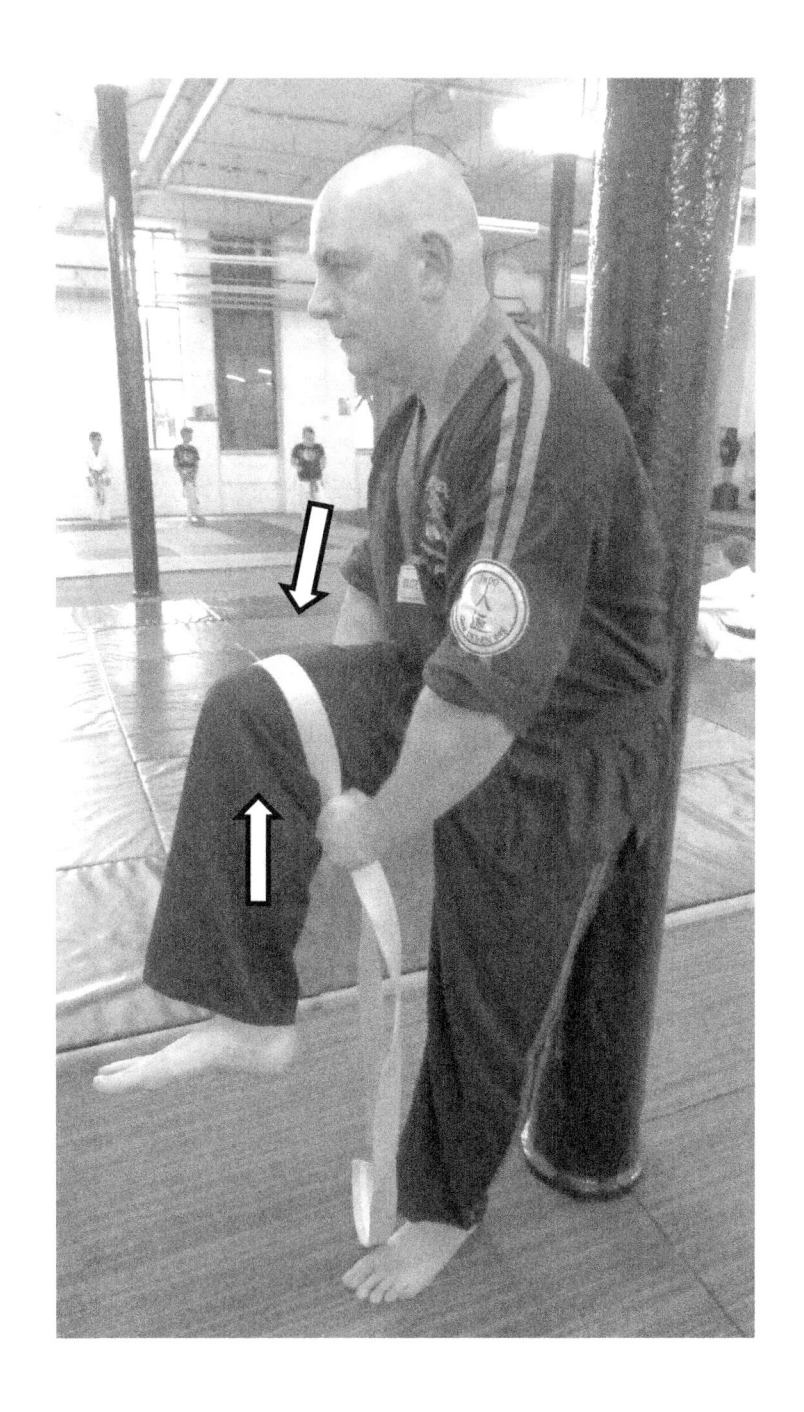

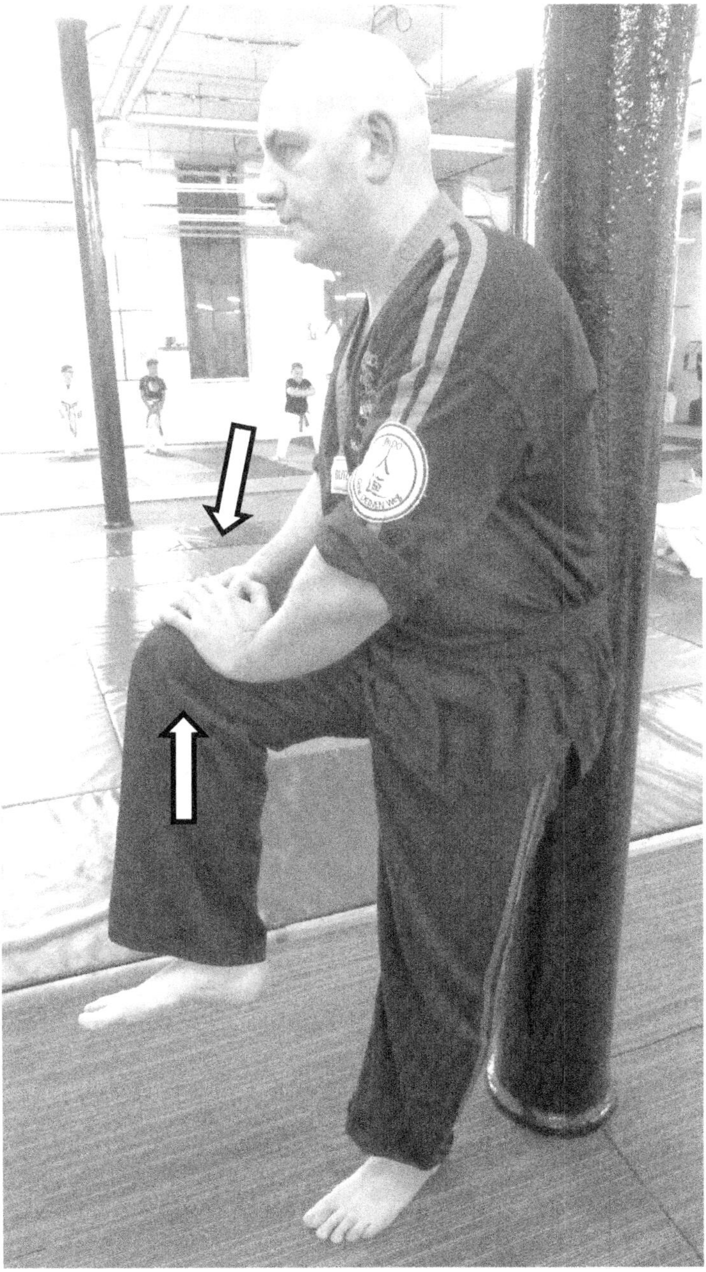

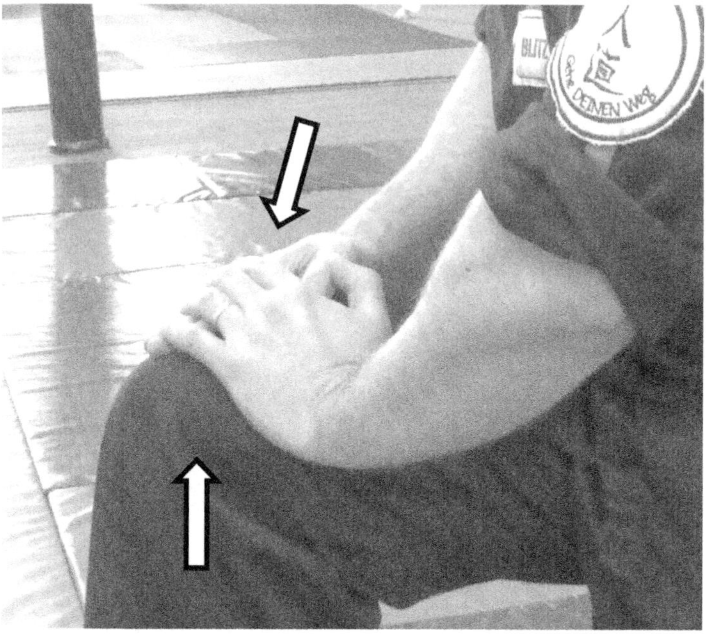
BLITZ
Gehe DEINEN Weg

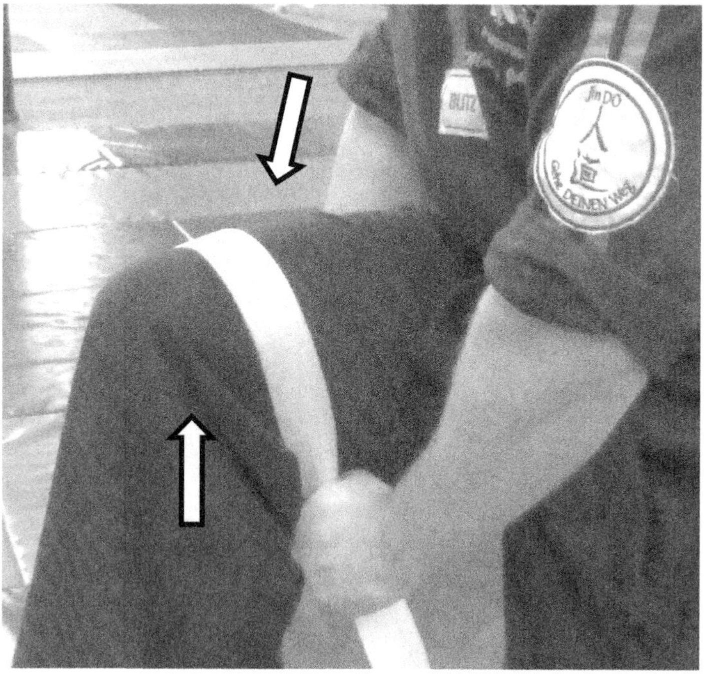
BLITZ
jin DO
Gehe DEINEN Weg

Abdominals – Oblique Trunk Twist

Stand upright in a forward stance. It does not matter if it is a left or right stance as you will exercise both sides of the body when one exercise is completed by changing to the other leg etc. Hold an unfurled martial arts belt, or similar, in both hands and with it looped under the leading foot. Start with the torso facing forward, but then twist back to the side holding the longer section of the belt.

Make sure that the belt is only long enough to stop you from fully twisting to the side and back so that you are at about the halfway position when you perform the exercise. Use the oblique abdominal muscles and the muscles of the hip and lower back to drive the exercise. Be sure to exercise both sides of the body by changing sides etc. The harder you engage the muscles, the more intense the exercise becomes, so always be sure to exercise at an intensity that best suits your current ability. When you perform an isometric exercise never hold your breath. Always breathe deeply and naturally, which will be about 10 full breaths in and out at a rate of about 1 second per full breath. Perform each exercise for no less than 7 seconds, and no longer than 10.

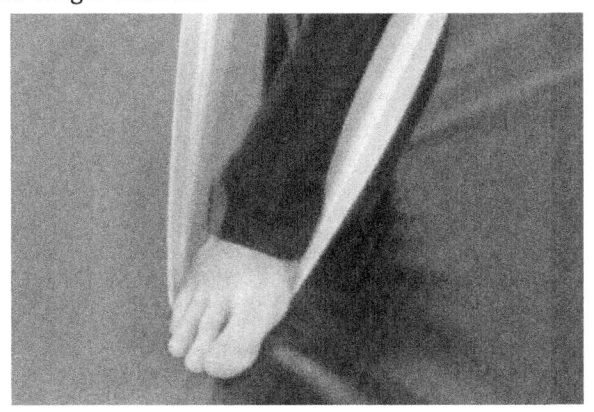

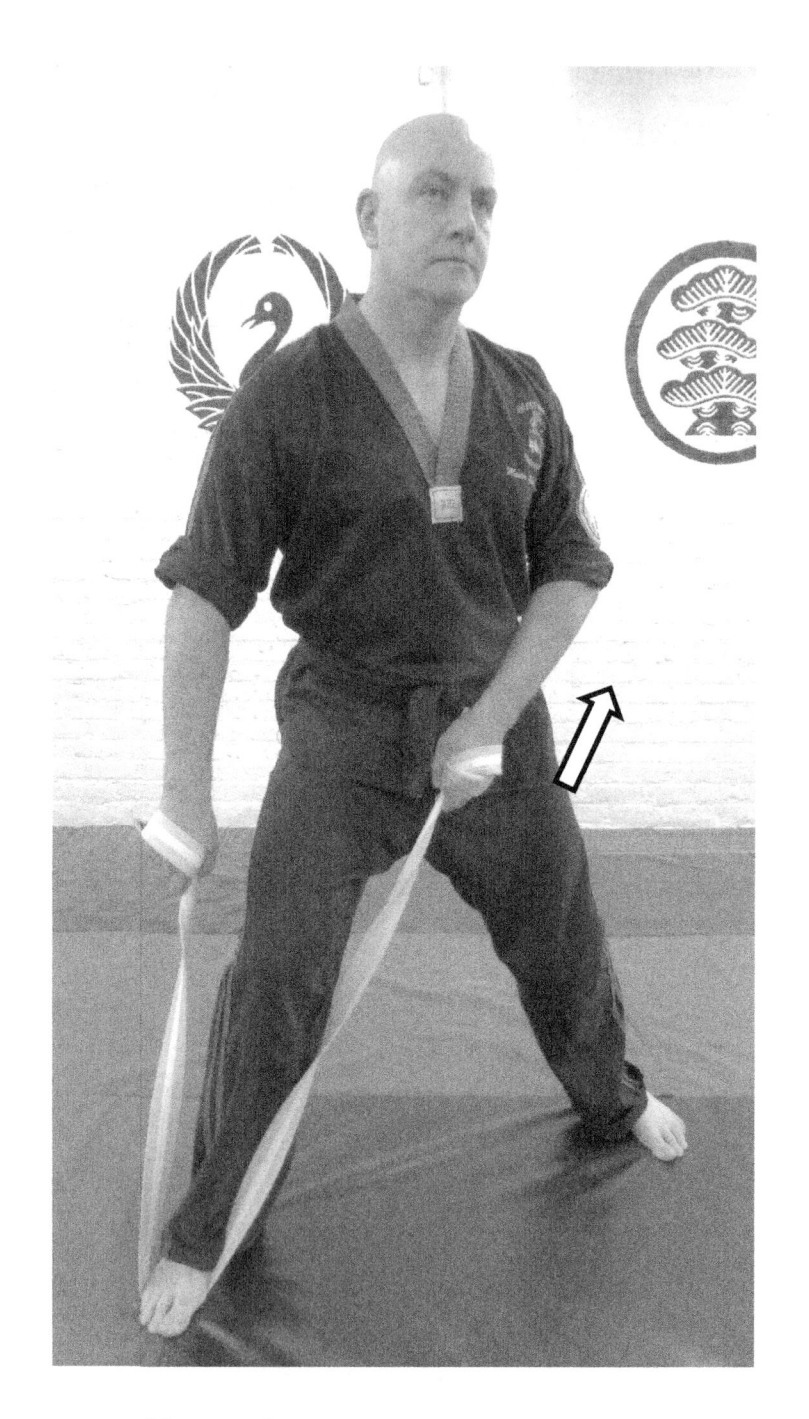

Abdominals – Standing Side Bend

Stand upright with your feet approximately shoulder-width apart. Place an unfurled martial arts belt under both feet at approximately equal length and hold each end, one in each hand.

Keep your hips straight and aligned in the neutral position. Bend slightly to one side using the provide the limiting position where you will perform the isometric exercise as you attempt to bend further but are prevented from doing so by the other hand gripping the belt which forms a loop under your feet. Be sure to exercise both sides of the body by changing sides etc.

The harder you engage the muscles, the more intense the exercise becomes, so always be sure to exercise at an intensity that best suits your current ability. When you perform an isometric exercise never hold your breath.

Always breathe deeply and naturally, which will be about 10 full breaths in and out at a rate of about 1 second per full breath. Perform each exercise for no less than 7 seconds, and no longer than 10.

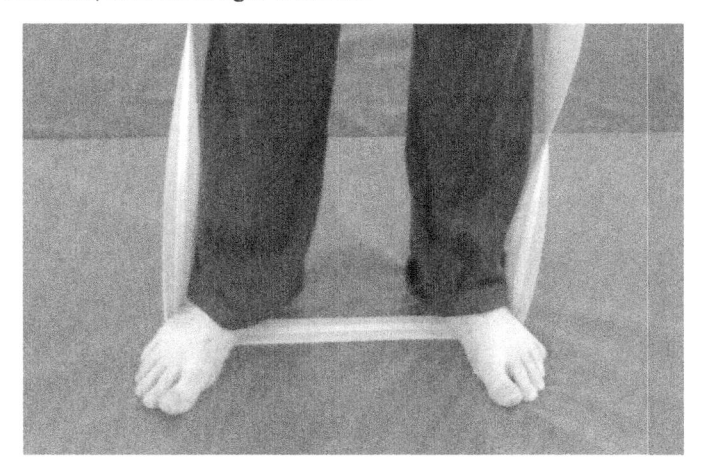

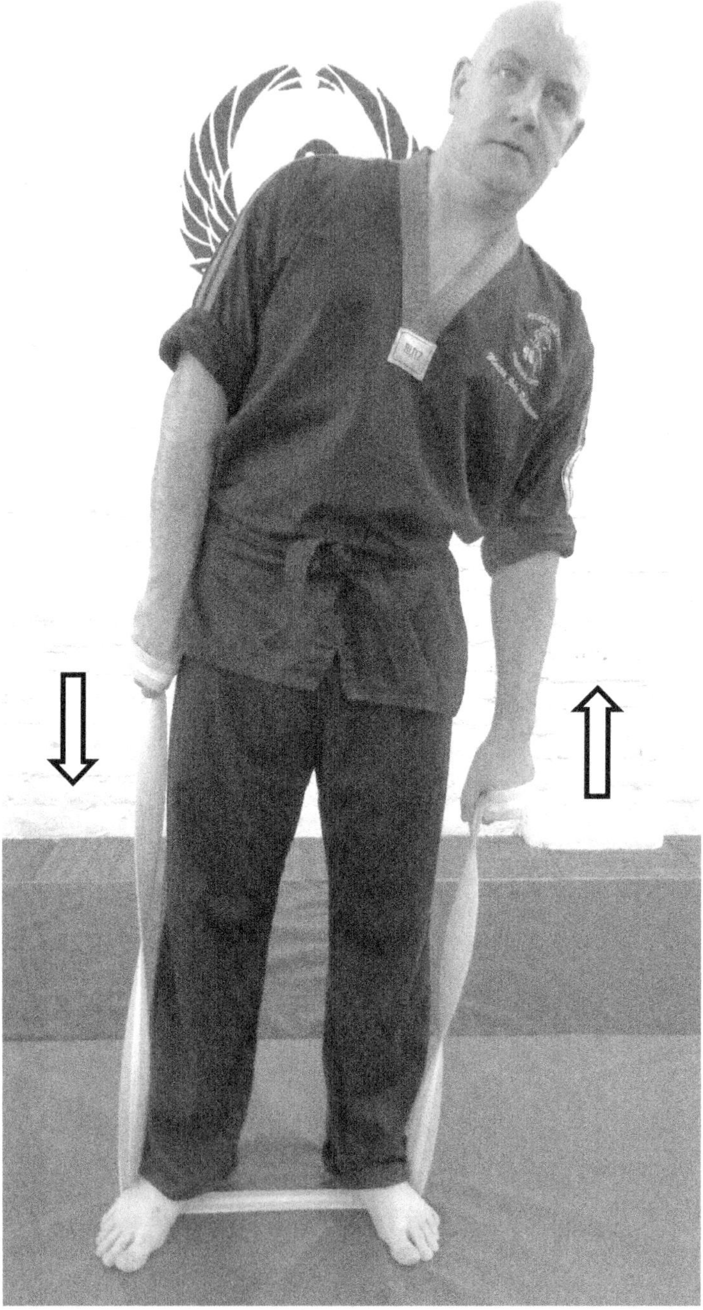

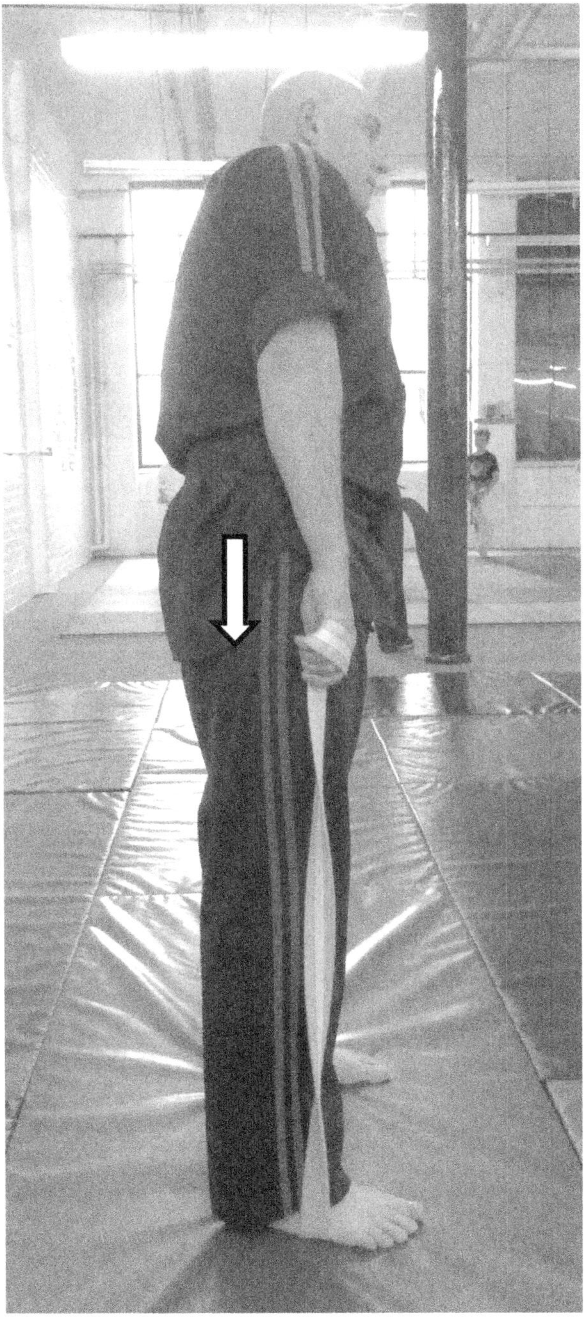

Abdominals – Kneeling Side Bend

Kneel on a mat upright with your knees approximately shoulder-width apart. Place an unfurled martial arts belt under both knees at approximately equal length and hold each end, one in each hand.

Keep your hips straight and aligned in the neutral position. Bend slightly to one side using the provide the limiting position where you will perform the isometric exercise as you attempt to bend further but are prevented from doing so by the other hand gripping the belt which forms a loop under your knees. Be sure to exercise both sides of the body by changing sides etc.

The harder you engage the muscles, the more intense the exercise becomes, so always be sure to exercise at an intensity that best suits your current ability. When you perform an isometric exercise never hold your breath. Always breathe deeply and naturally, which will be about 10 full breaths in and out at a rate of about 1 second per full breath. Perform each exercise for no less than 7 seconds, and no longer than 10.

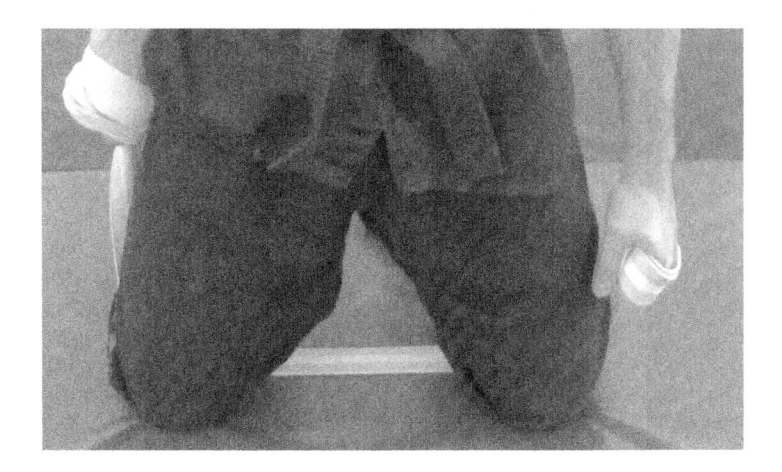

105

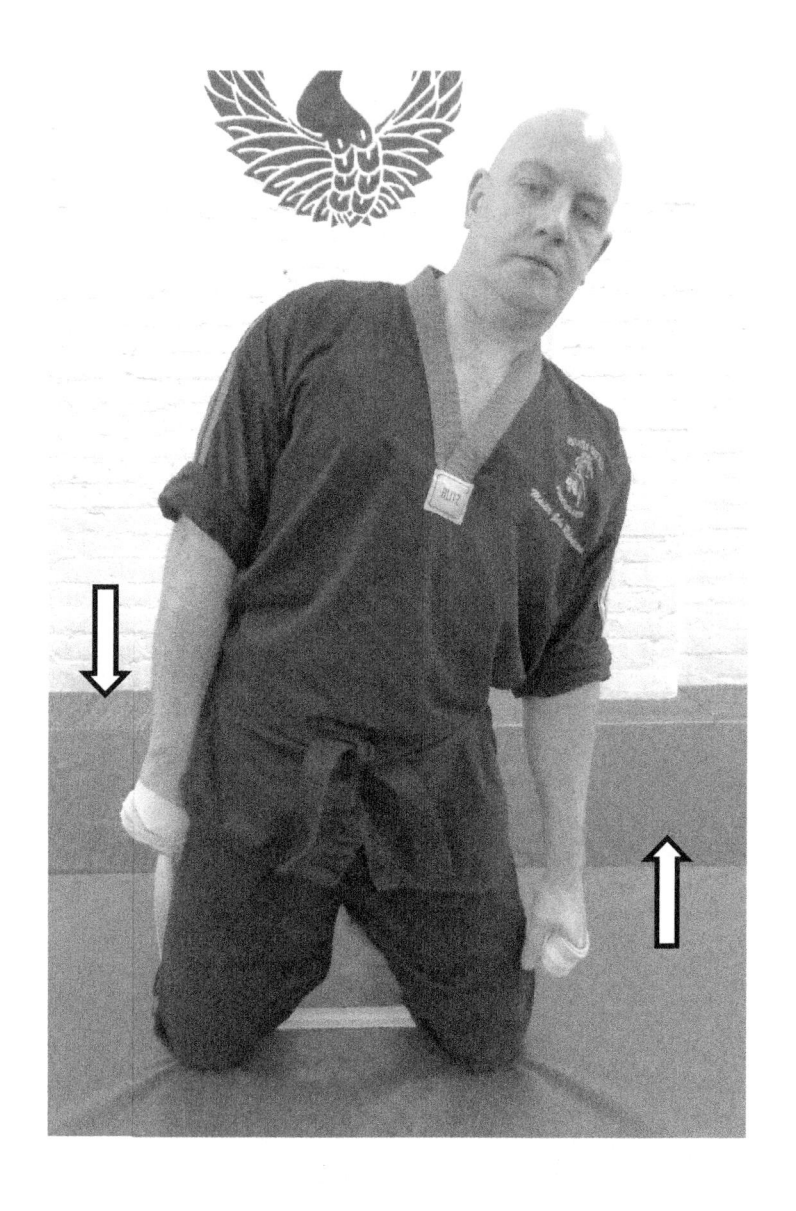

106

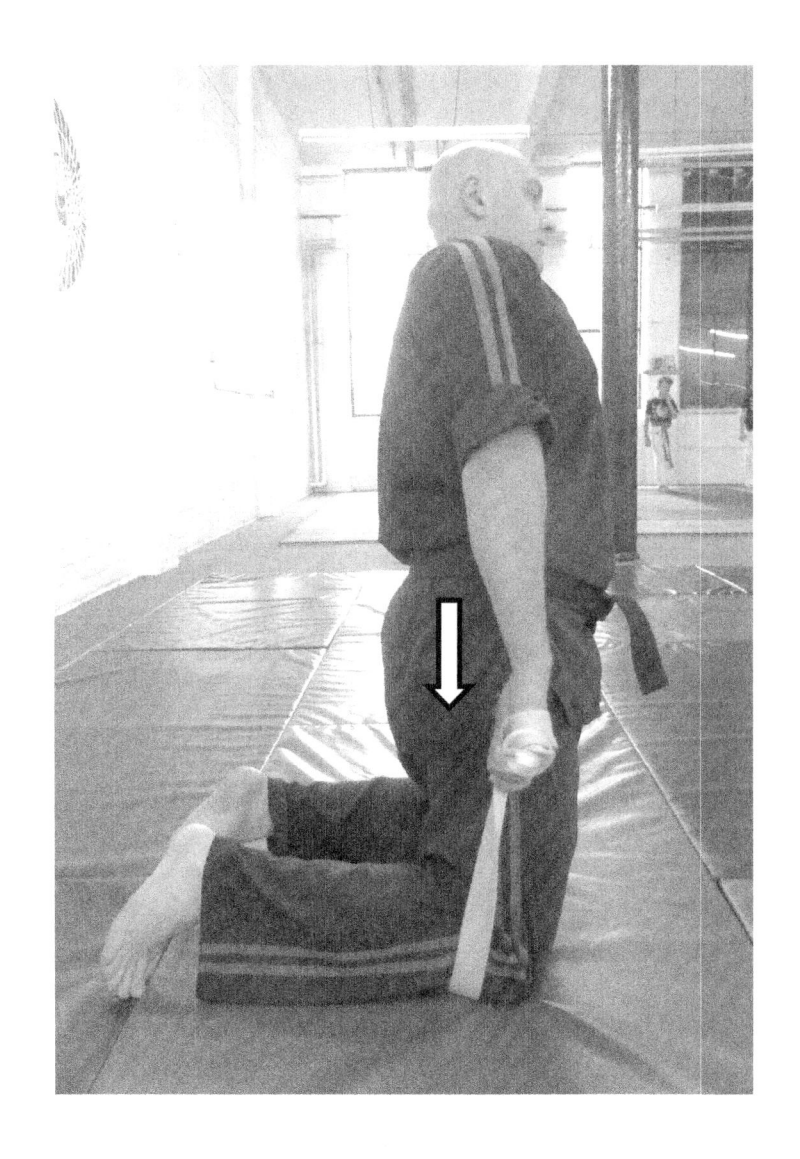

Arms – Biceps Upright Belt Curl

Stand upright in a forward stance. It does not matter if it is a left or right stance. Loop and unfurled martial arts belt, or similar, under the forward foot, and hold each of the other ends one in each hand.

Make sure that the length of the belt looped around each hand is enough to allow you to bend both of your arms to an approximately equal midpoint. In this position, engage the biceps muscles to perform a biceps curl

The harder you engage the muscles, the more intense the exercise becomes, so always be sure to exercise at an intensity that best suits your current ability. When you perform an isometric exercise never hold your breath.

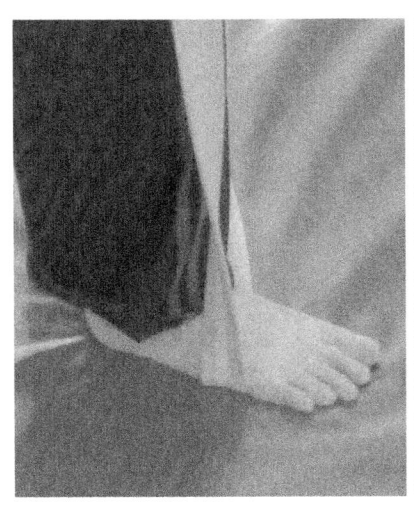

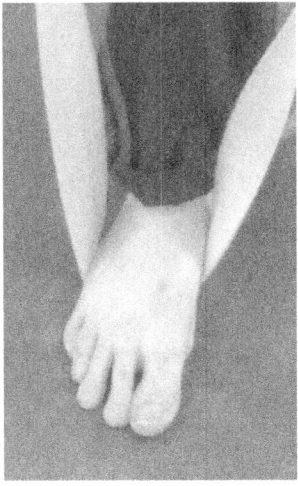

Always breathe deeply and naturally, which will be about 10 full breaths in and out at a rate of about 1 second per full breath. Perform each exercise for no less than 7 seconds, and no longer than 10.

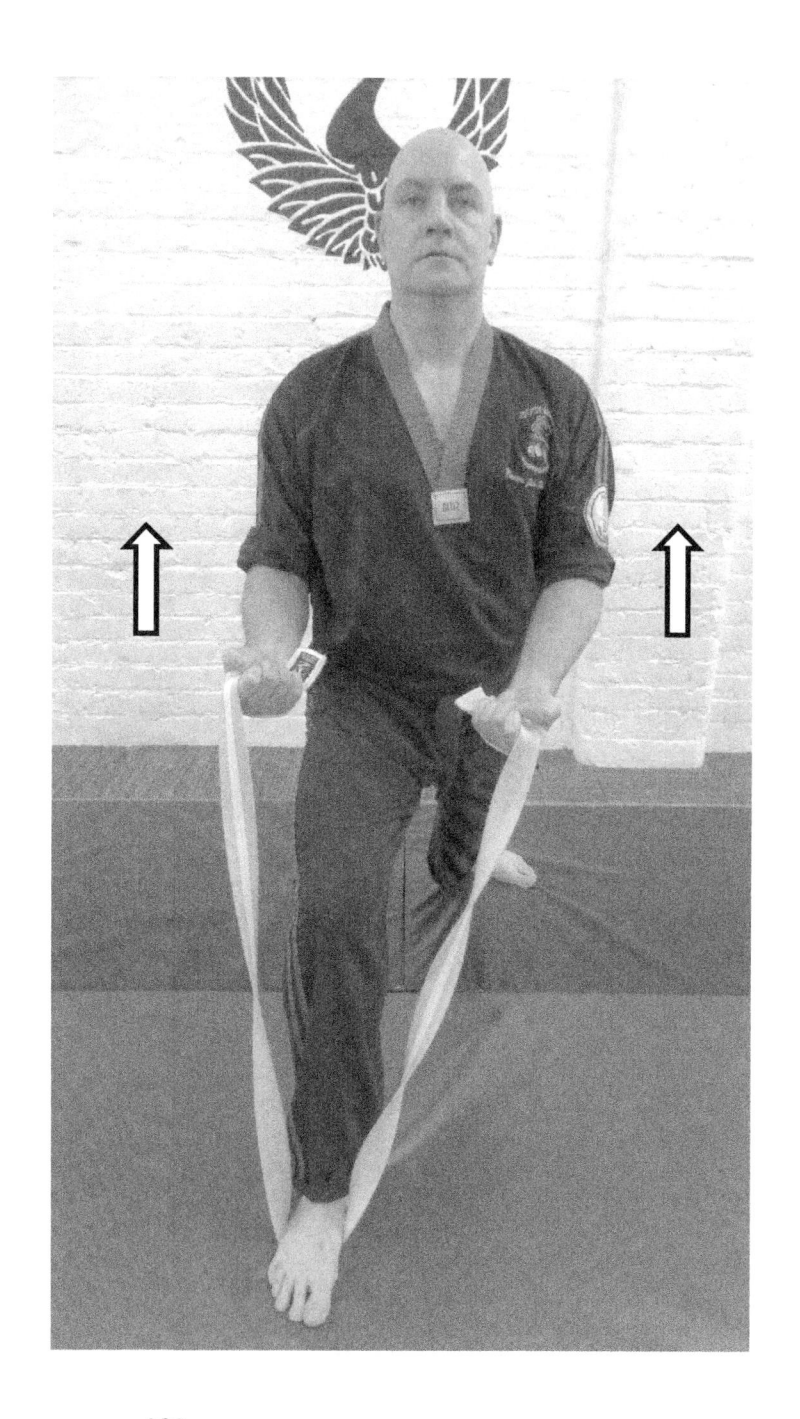

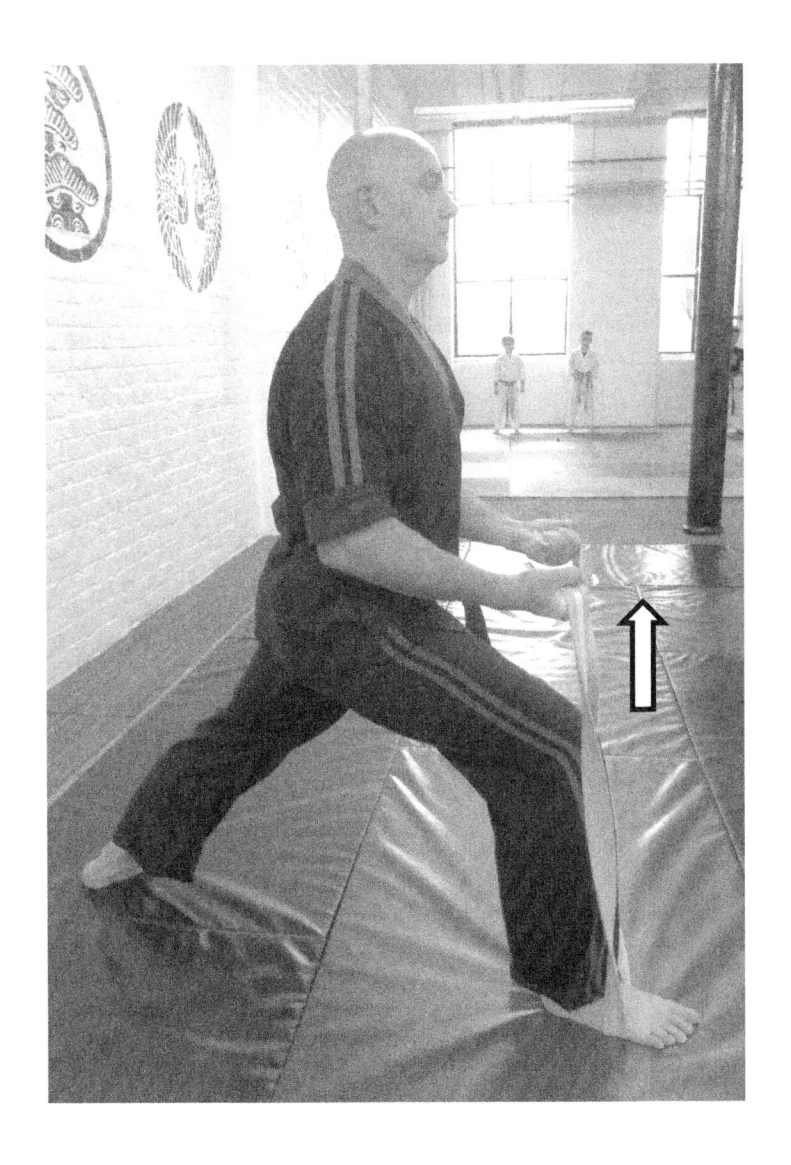

Arms – Biceps Thumbs-up Belt Curl

Stand upright with an unfurled martial arts belt under one foot. This can be secured either by gripping each end of the belt one in each hand or by gripping both sides of the belt in one hand to perform the exercise.

Loop the belt around the hand with sufficient length to allow you to perform an approximate midpoint biceps isometric curl with your thumbs upright and your little finger to the bottom. Be sure to exercise both sides of the body by changing sides etc.

in a forward stance. It does not matter if it is a left or right stance. Loop and unfurled martial arts belt, or similar, under the forward foot, and hold each of the other ends one in each hand.

Make sure that the length of the belt looped around each hand is enough to allow you to bend both of your arms to an approximately equal midpoint. In this position, engage the biceps muscles to perform a biceps curl.

The harder you engage the muscles, the more intense the exercise becomes, so always be sure to exercise at an intensity that best suits your current ability. When you perform an isometric exercise never hold your breath.

Always breathe deeply and naturally, which will be about 10 full breaths in and out at a rate of about 1 second per full breath. Perform each exercise for no less than 7 seconds, and no longer than 10.

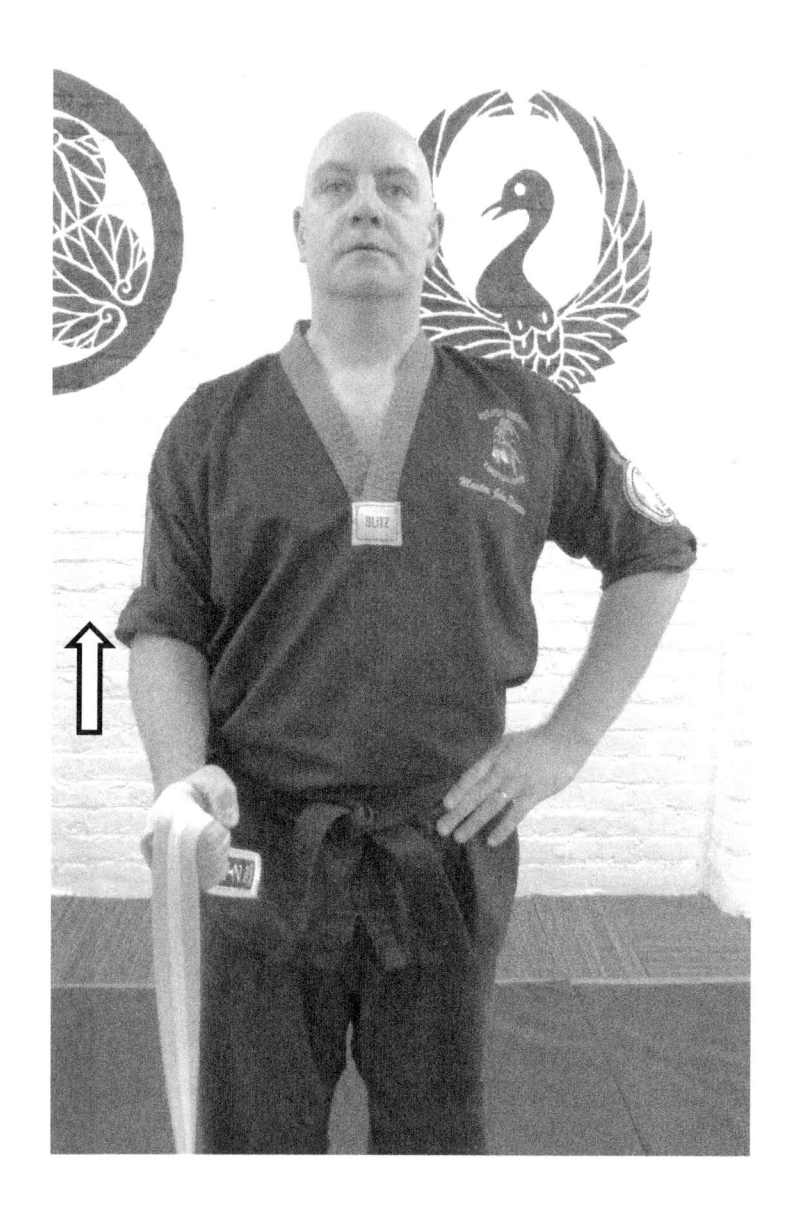

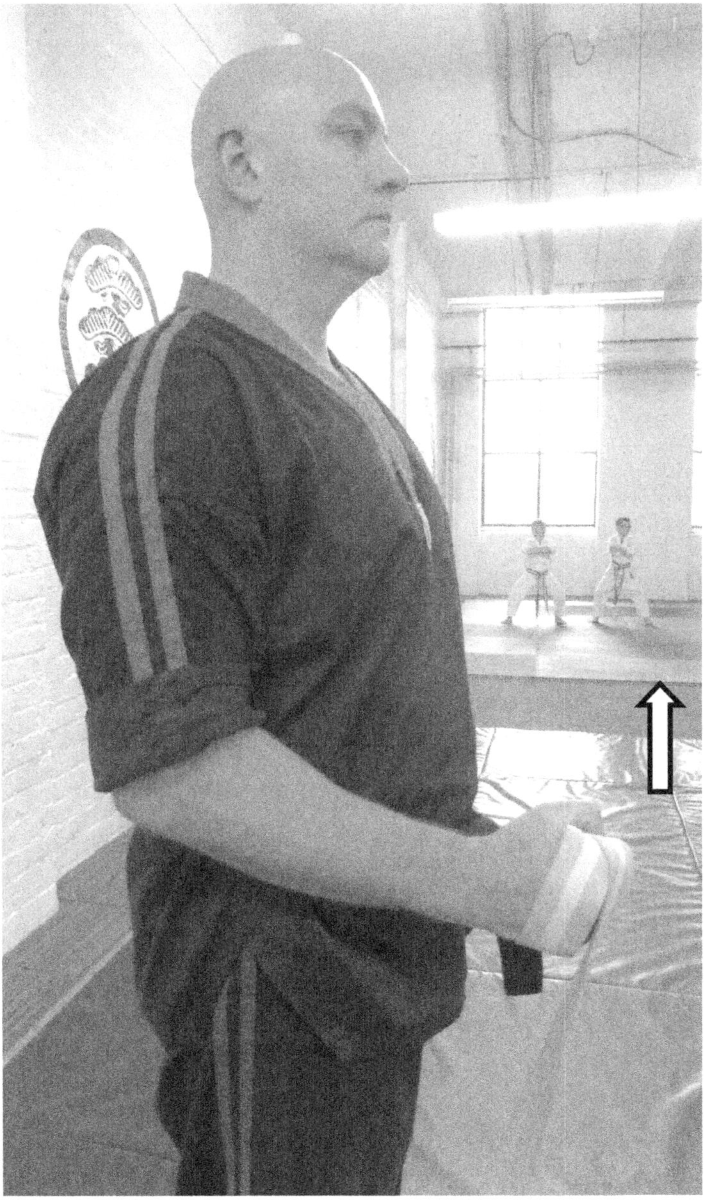

Arms – Biceps Under Thigh Belt Curl

Stand upright leaning back against a solid object such as a wall etc. Lift one leg with a bent knee. Loop an unfurled martial arts belt under the thigh close to the knee. Grip this with each end of the belt in each hand. Allow sufficient length to loop around the hand so that you can bend the arms to the approximate midpoint position. Apply force as if to raise the leg which resists the upward biceps curl action with the weight of the leg and also by pressing down with your thigh to counterbalance the curling action. When you have reached the desired point, perform the isometric exercise. The harder you engage the muscles, the more intense the exercise becomes, so always be sure to exercise at an intensity that best suits your current ability. When you perform an isometric exercise never hold your breath. Always breathe deeply and naturally, which will be about 10 full breaths in and out at a rate of about 1 second per full breath. Perform each exercise for no less than 7 seconds, and no longer than 10.

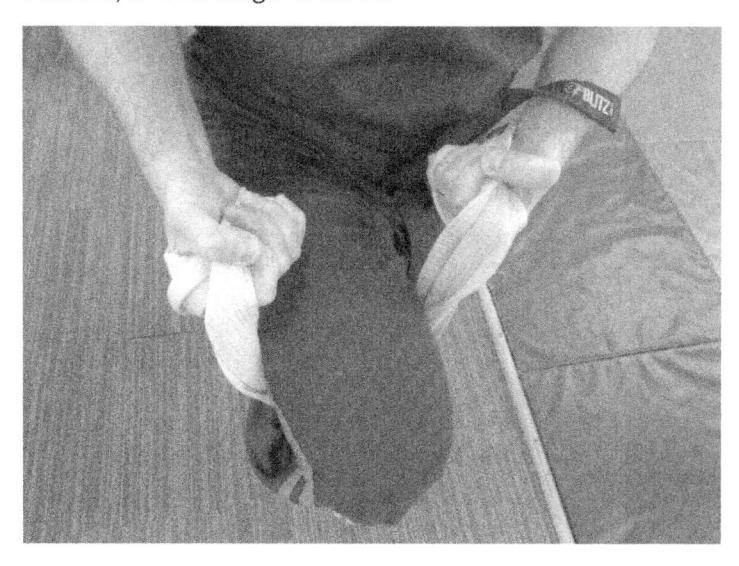

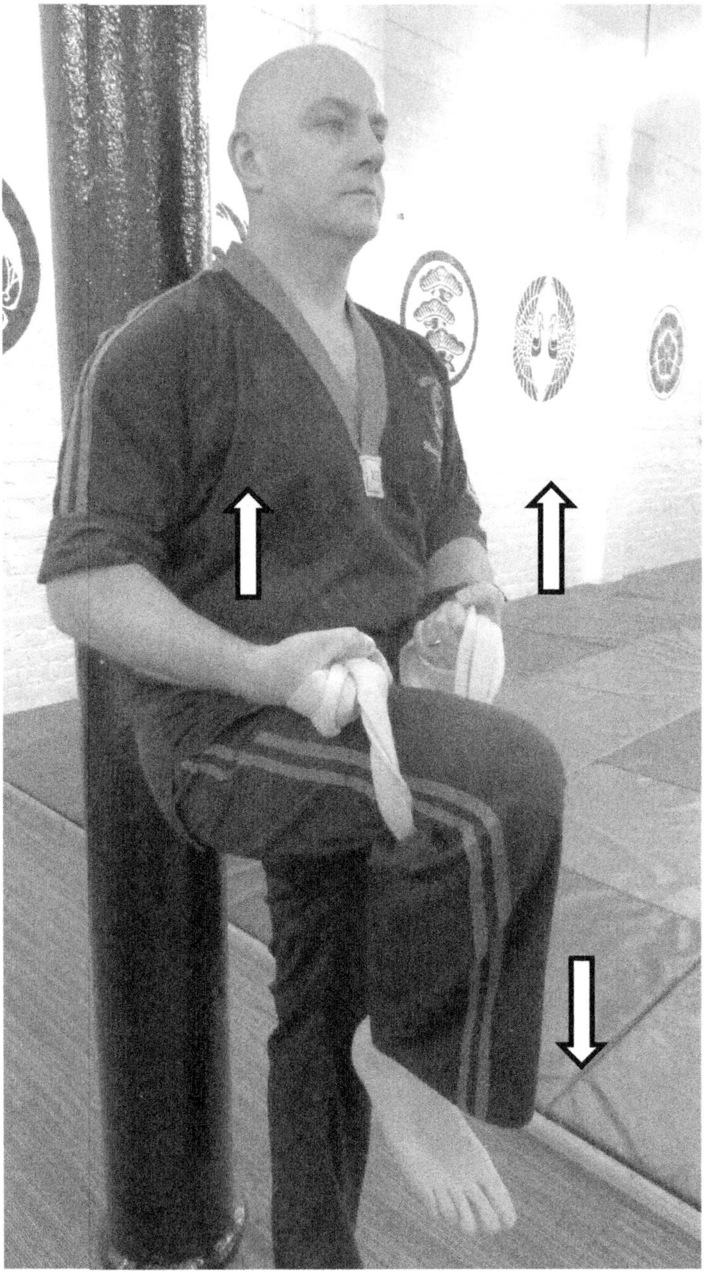

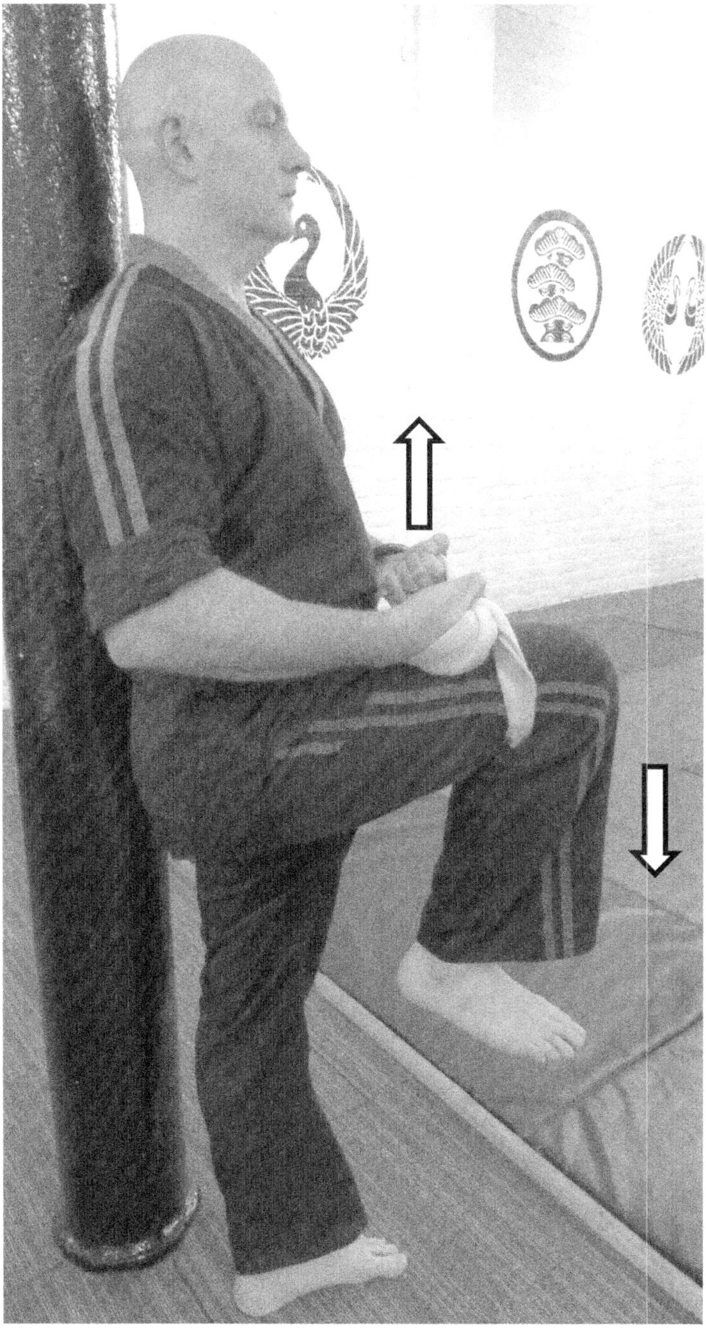

Arms – Biceps-Triceps Partner Curl-Press

The Upper arm biceps-triceps exercise engages both the front and rear upper arms. The exercise is in two parts. One part exercises the front upper arm of one side of the body and simultaneously the rear upper arm of the other side. In simple terms, one partner holds both of their hands at approximately mid-level with their elbows bent at approximately 90 degrees.

One hand is facing upward, the other hand is facing downward. The other partner mirrors this position except that they have their hands in opposing directions so they can interlock hands. Exercise partners must stand face to face with each other so they can effectively interlock hands at the same height to perform the exercise.

Be sure to always keep the arms roughly bent at the midpoint with the elbows close to the body throughout the exercise. Always be sure that both partners exercise both arms/sides of the body equally in both directions. So, after a change of grip position and direction of effort, the emphasis of the exercise reverses for both partners.

The harder you engage the muscles, the more intense the exercise becomes, so always be sure to exercise at an intensity that best suits your current ability. When you perform an isometric exercise never hold your breath.

Always breathe deeply and naturally, which will be about 10 full breaths in and out at a rate of about 1 second per full breath. Perform each exercise for no less than 7 seconds, and no longer than 10.

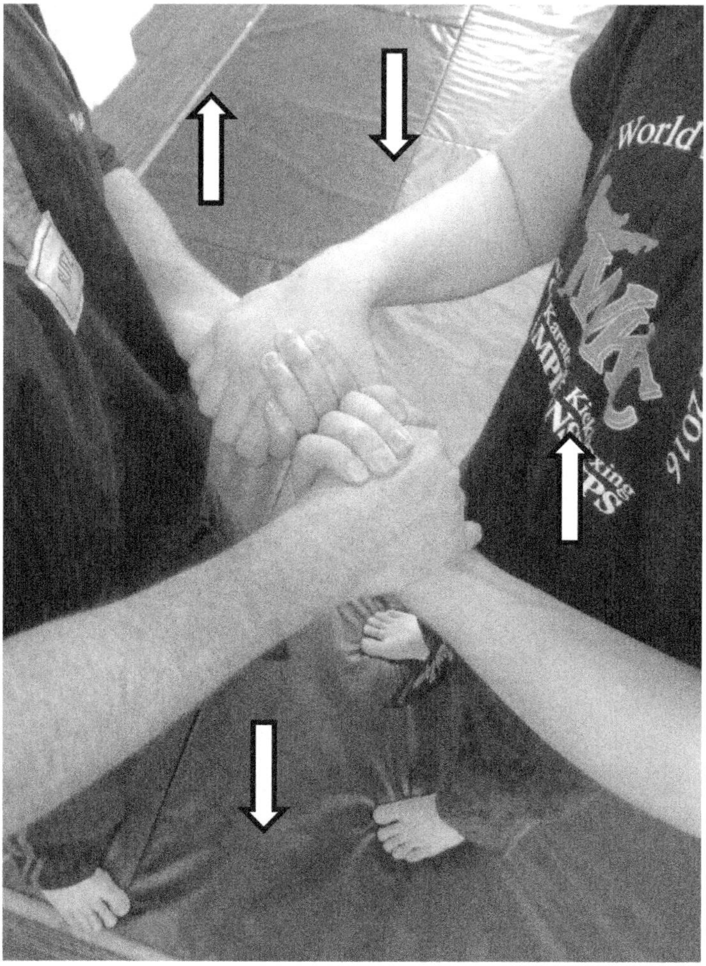
World

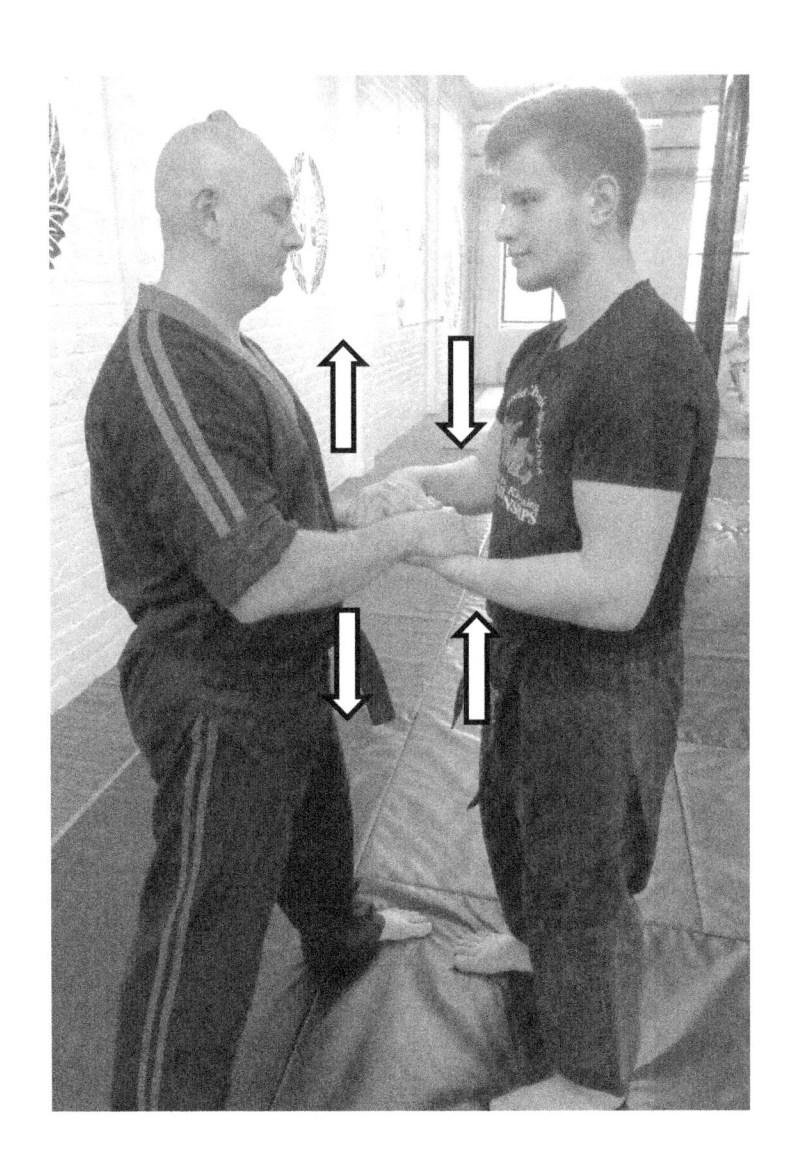

Biceps-Triceps Curl-Press Variation 1.

This variation is performed without the need for a partner. Simply interlock your left and right hands at the midpoint near the waist and close to the body. One hand attempts to curl the arm upward, and the other attempts to press the arm/hand down. The isometric exercise is performed in the same way as the partner exercise.

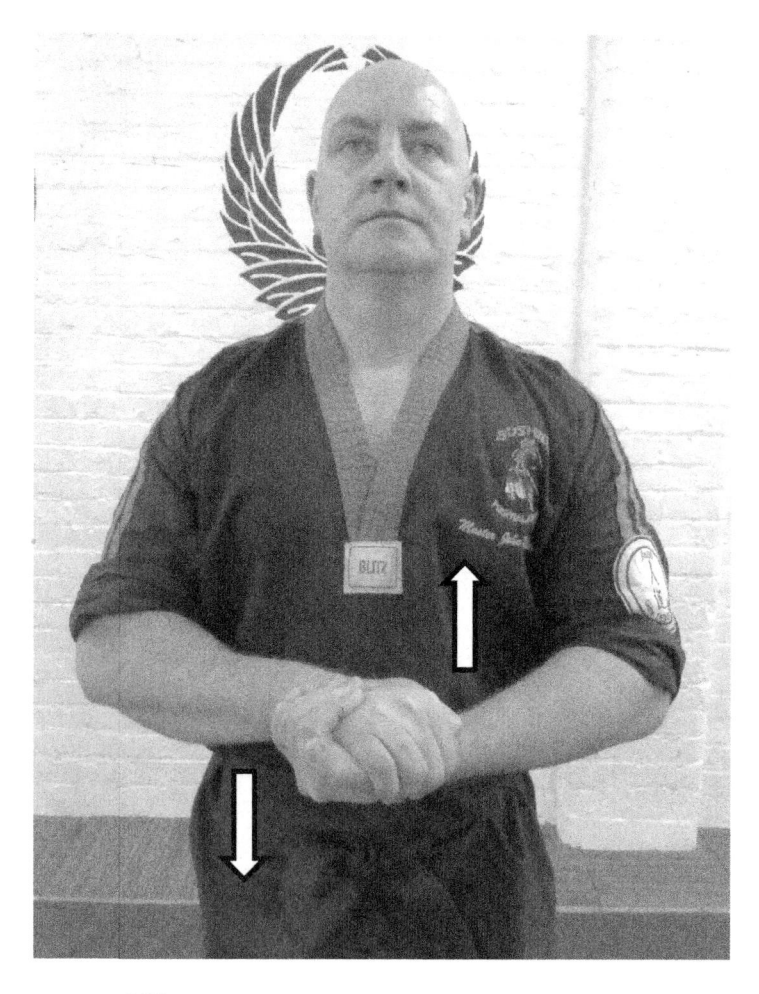

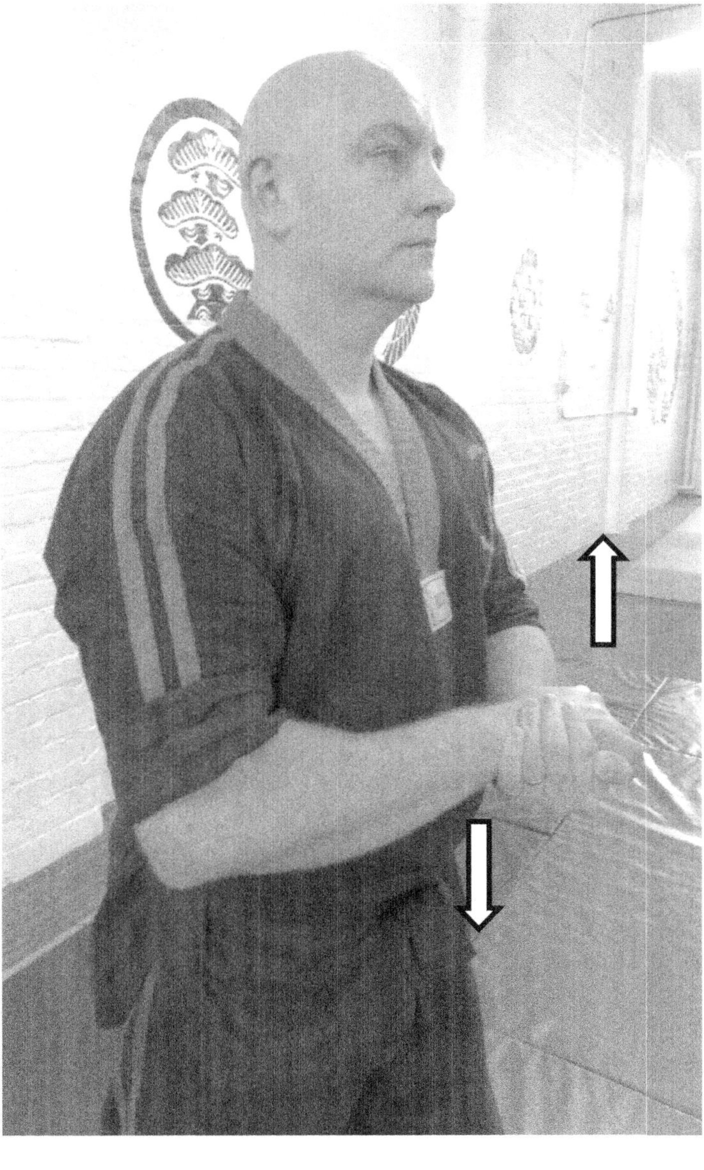

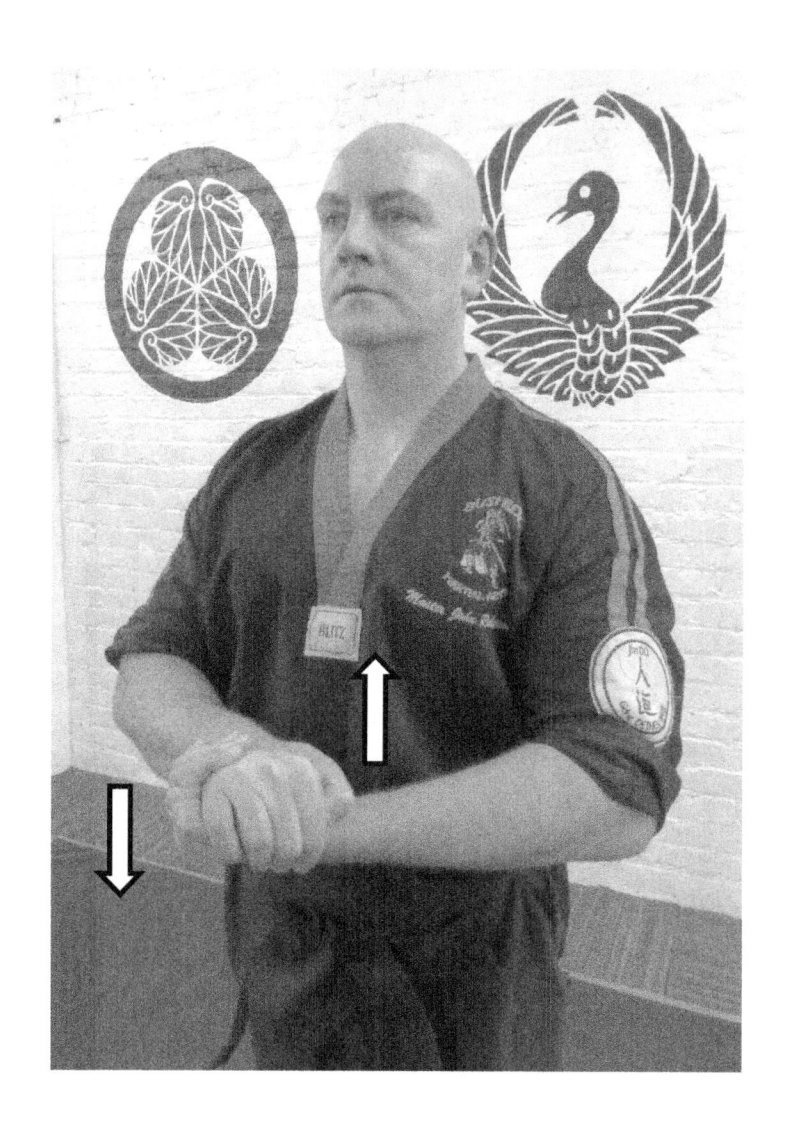

Biceps-Triceps Curl-Press Variation 2.

This variation is performed without the need for a partner. Instead of interlocking your hands, you use a martial arts belt looped around each hand. This method offers certain benefits that others do not. None is better or worse, they are all merely different and all are useful and valid exercises in their own right. One hand attempts to curl the arm upward, and the other hand attempts to press the arm/hand down. The isometric exercise is performed in the same way as the partner exercise.

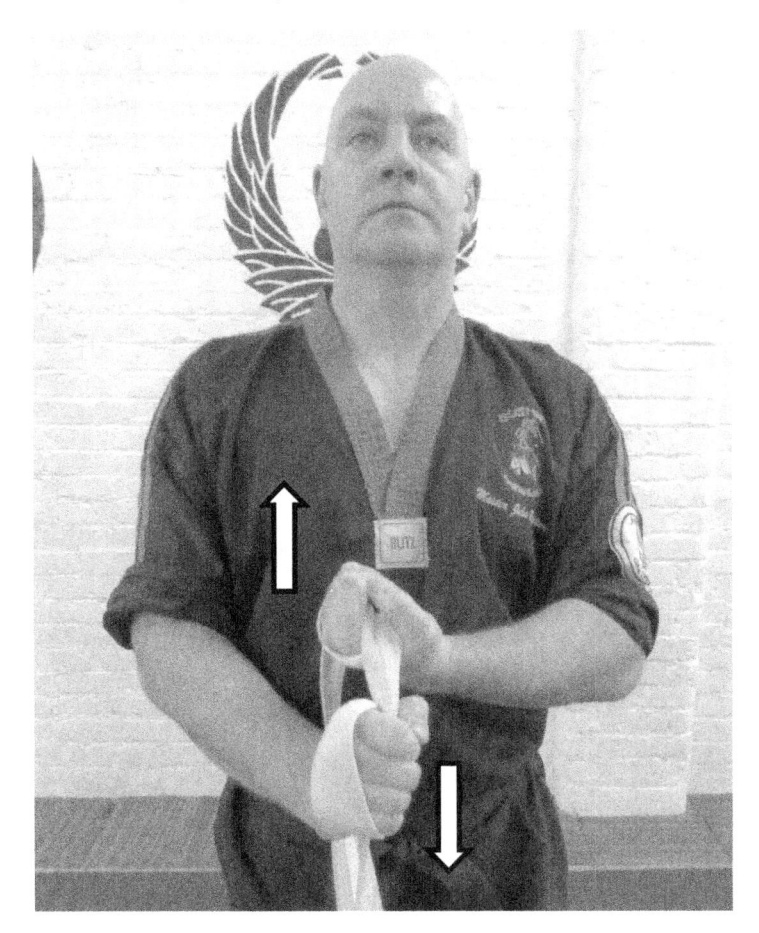

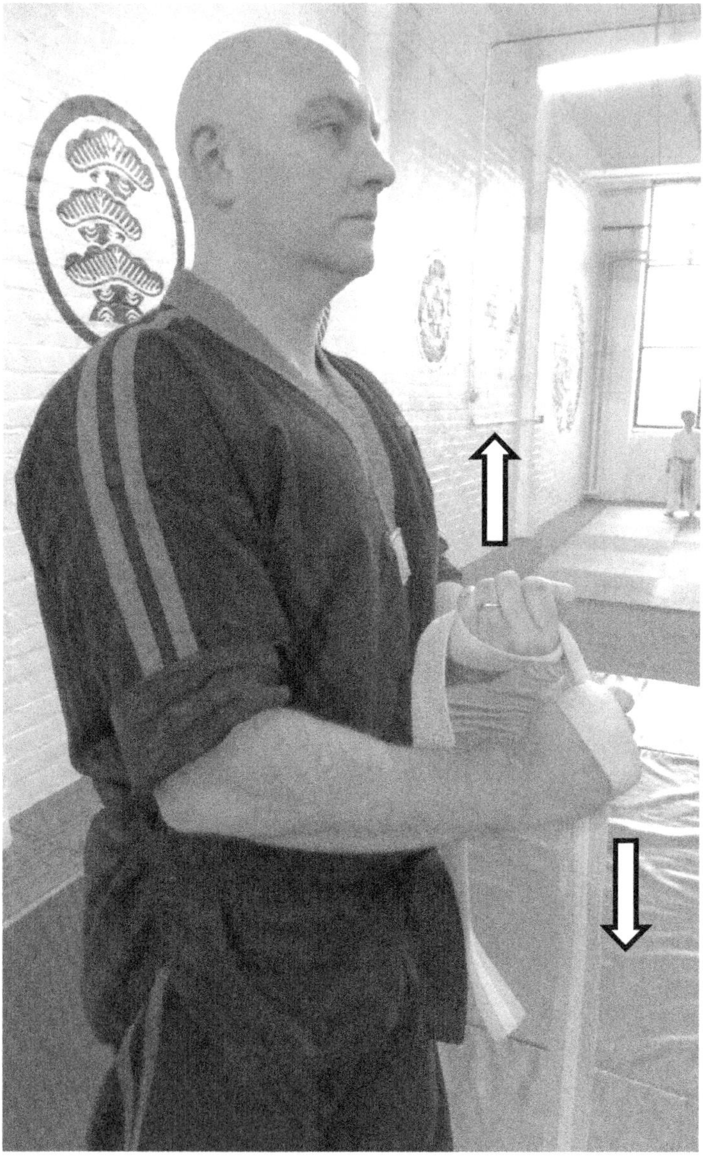

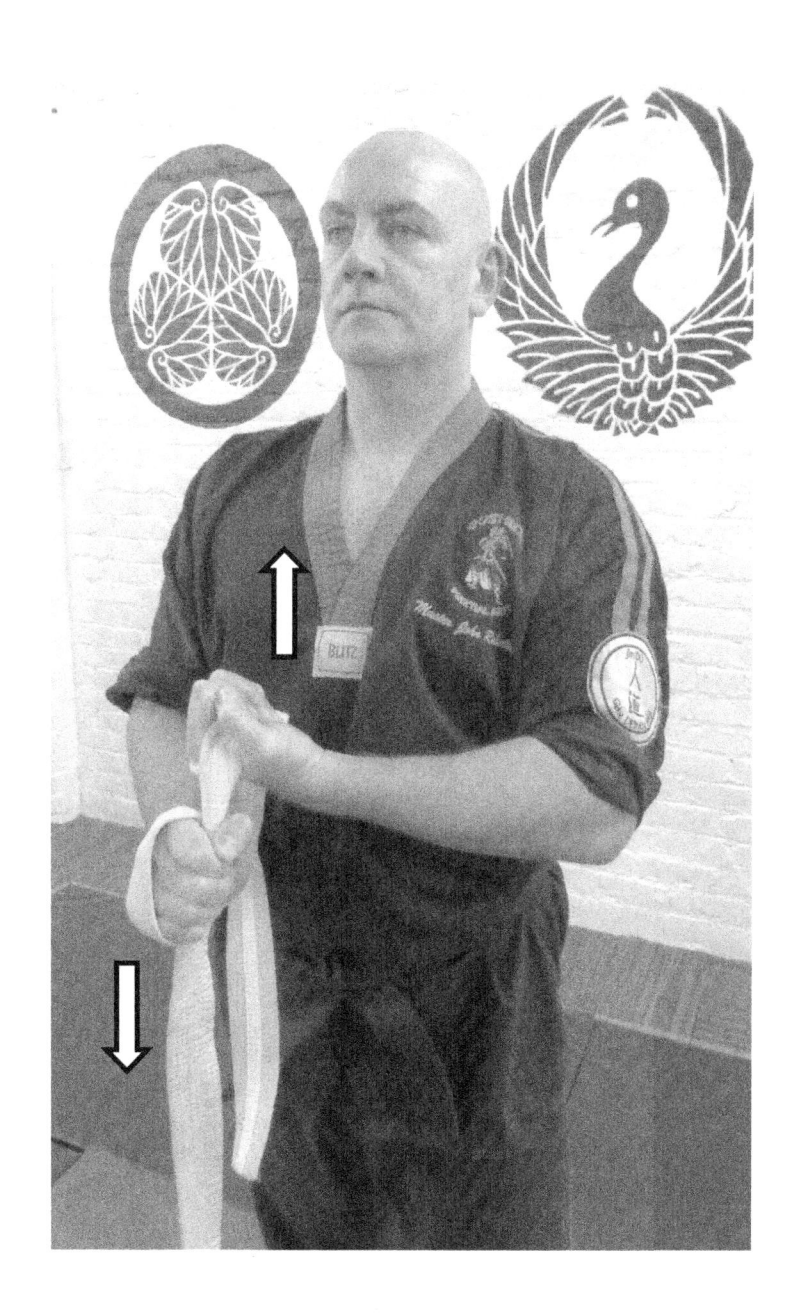

Arms – Forearms Water Bottle Grip

You will ideally need two plastic bottles with a screw cap. Fill both up to the brim with plain tap water and ensure there is no, or only a minimum air gap. Do not use a glass bottle, a can, or a plastic one filled with carbonated liquid as this may burst.

Stand upright and hold one bottle in each hand, with your hands and arms slightly away from the body. In this position, apply as much force with your grip as you try to compress and crush the bottle. Since water cannot be compressed, it will perfectly counterbalance even the strongest grip that is applied.

This exercise is even better if two additional bottles of different diameters are prepared in the same way to exercise the grip in a different position.

The harder you engage the muscles, the more intense the exercise becomes, so always be sure to exercise at an intensity that best suits your current ability. When you perform an isometric exercise never hold your breath.

Always breathe deeply and naturally, which will be about 10 full breaths in and out at a rate of about 1 second per full breath. Perform each exercise for no less than 7 seconds, and no longer than 10.

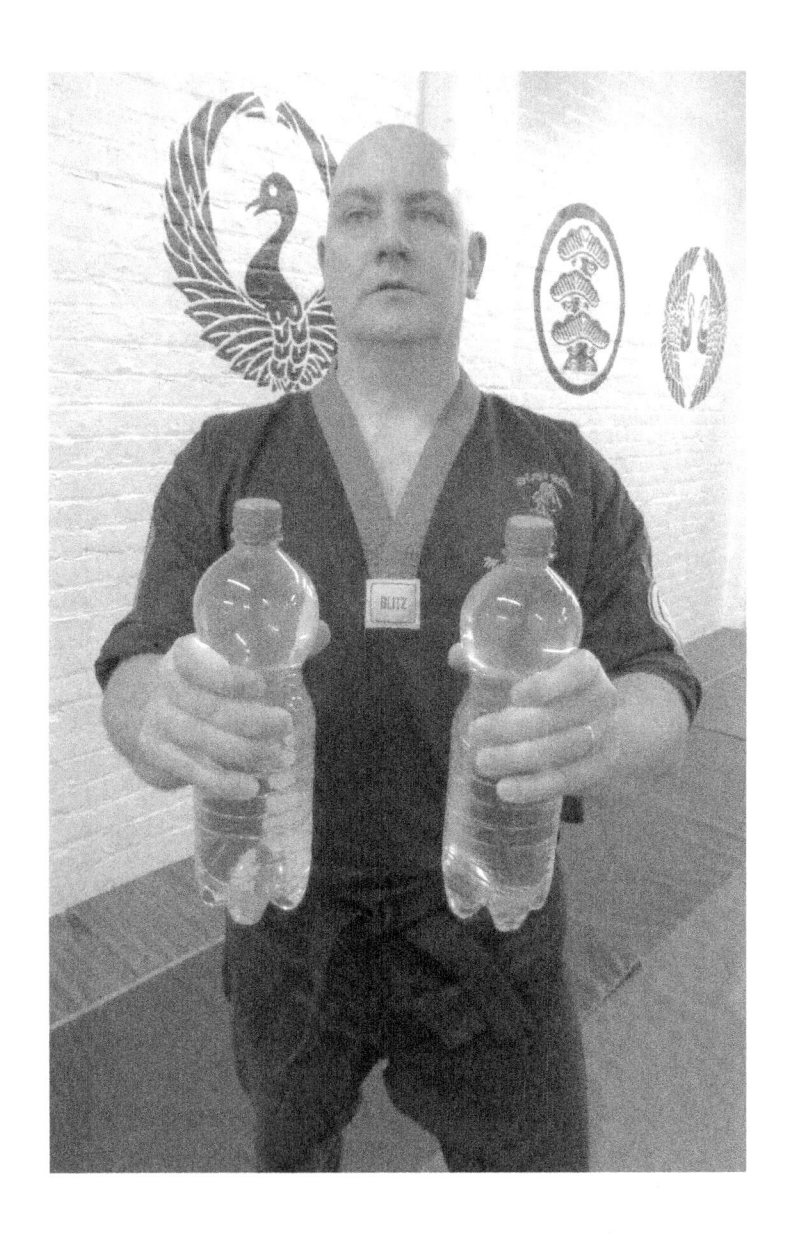

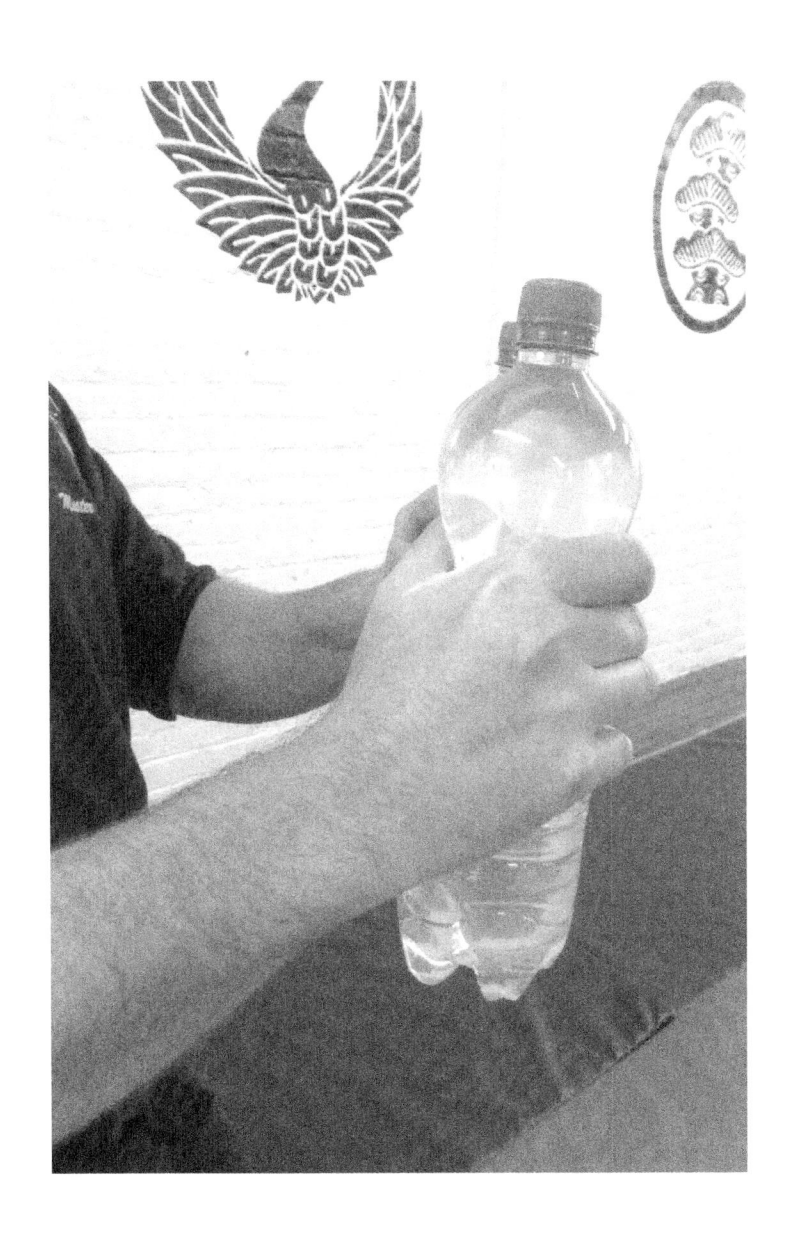

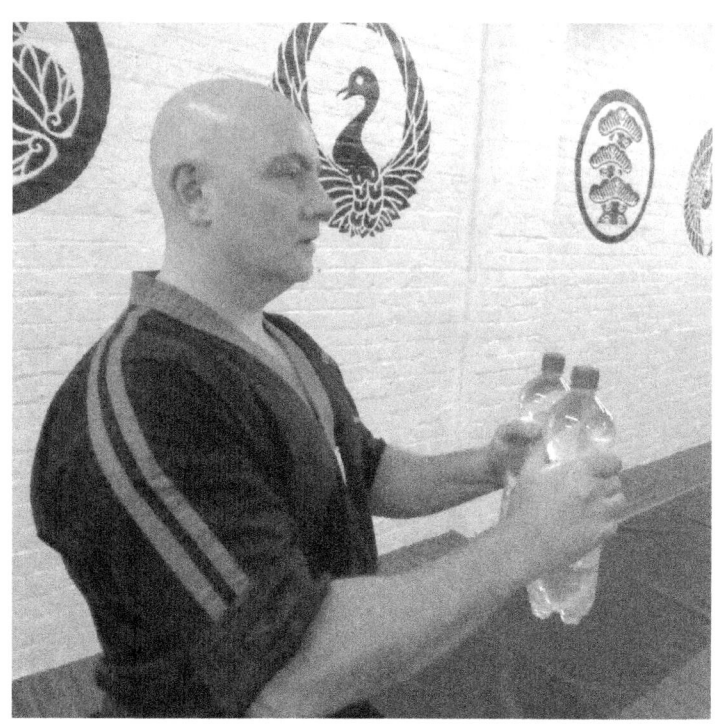

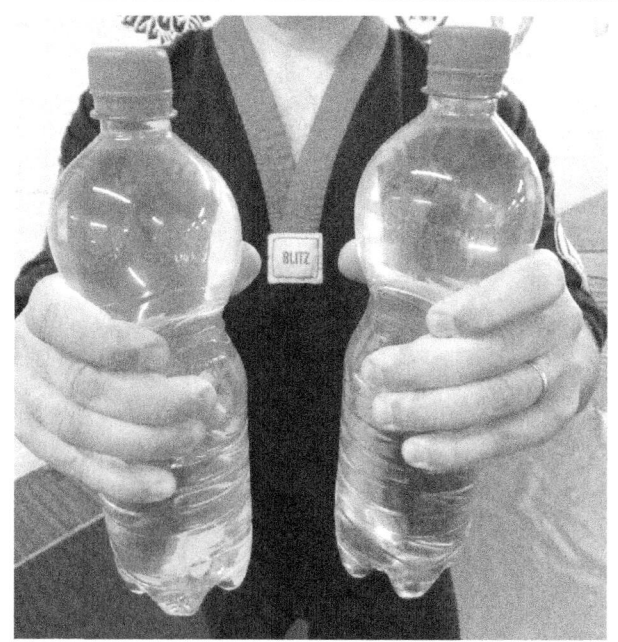

Arms – Triceps Side Extension Backfist

Stand upright with one arm held out to the side so that it is horizontal to the floor and with the elbow bent. Hold an unfurled martial arts belt in your hand so that it is looped around it so that you are in the back fist strike position. Hold the other end of the martial arts belt in the other hand and secure it at approximately chest height with your elbow bent. In this position, apply force outward and to the side as if attempting to slowly perform the back-fist strike movement until you reach the midpoint position to perform the isometric exercise in. Be sure to exercise both sides of the body by changing sides etc. The harder you engage the muscles, the more intense the exercise becomes, so always be sure to exercise at an intensity that best suits your current ability. When you perform an isometric exercise never hold your breath. Always breathe deeply and naturally, which will be about 10 full breaths in and out at a rate of about 1 second per full breath. Perform each exercise for no less than 7 seconds, and no longer than 10.

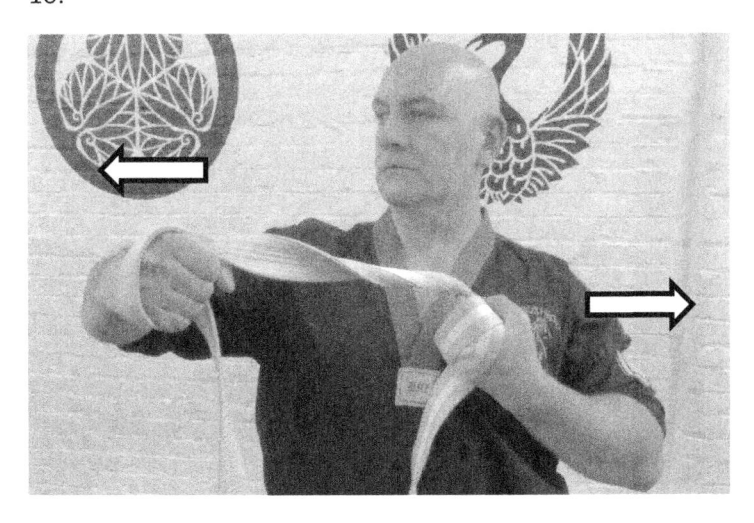

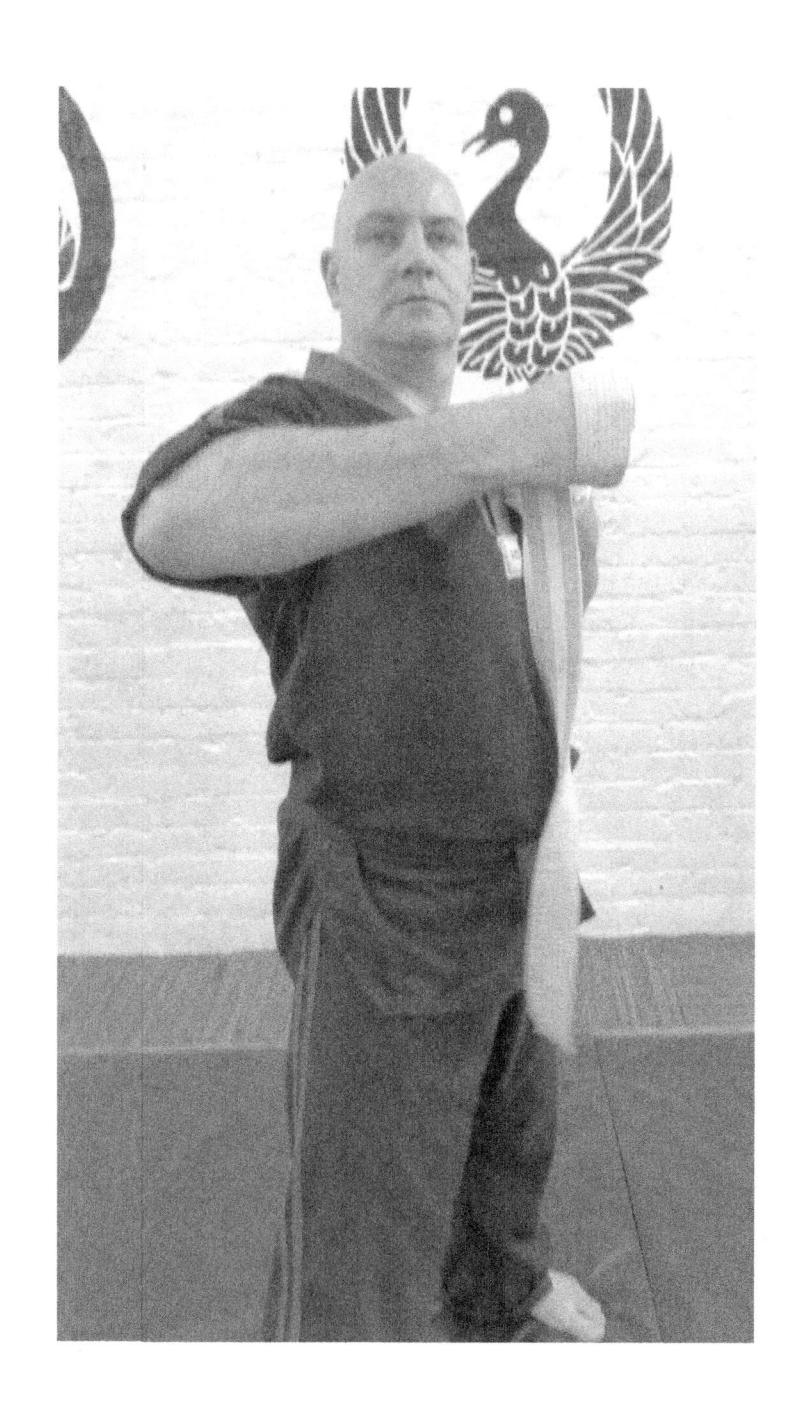

Arms – Triceps Front Press

Lie face down flat on an exercise mat on the floor. Place both arms and elbows tucked under you and close to the body with your palms facing down flat to touch the floor just under the front of your shoulders. Pressing forward and downwards, engage the triceps muscles to push yourself up so that your arms are bent at the approximate midpoint between the floor and completely upright. This is when you can begin the isometric exercise. The harder you engage the muscles, the more intense the exercise becomes, so always be sure to exercise at an intensity that best suits your current ability. When you perform an isometric exercise never hold your breath. Always breathe deeply and naturally, which will be about 10 full breaths in and out at a rate of about 1 second per full breath. Perform each exercise for no less than 7 seconds, and no longer than 10. **NOTE:** If you need to make the exercise easier, simply drop down from suspending your body on your hands and feet, to perform the exercise from your hands and knees instead. The more acute the angle of your elbows, the harder the exercise will be, and the more obtuse the elbow angle, the easier the exercise will be. Similarly, the closer the hands are together the harder the exercise will be, and the wider the hand position, to a maximum of shoulder-width apart, the easier the exercise will be. Performing the exercise starting with a close hand position, the forearms flat on the floor and with the most acute elbow angle will be the hardest way. The easiest way will be with a shoulder-width apart hand spacing and most obtuse elbow angle, starting from the upper position and then lowering to a point before your forearms come to rest flat on the floor.

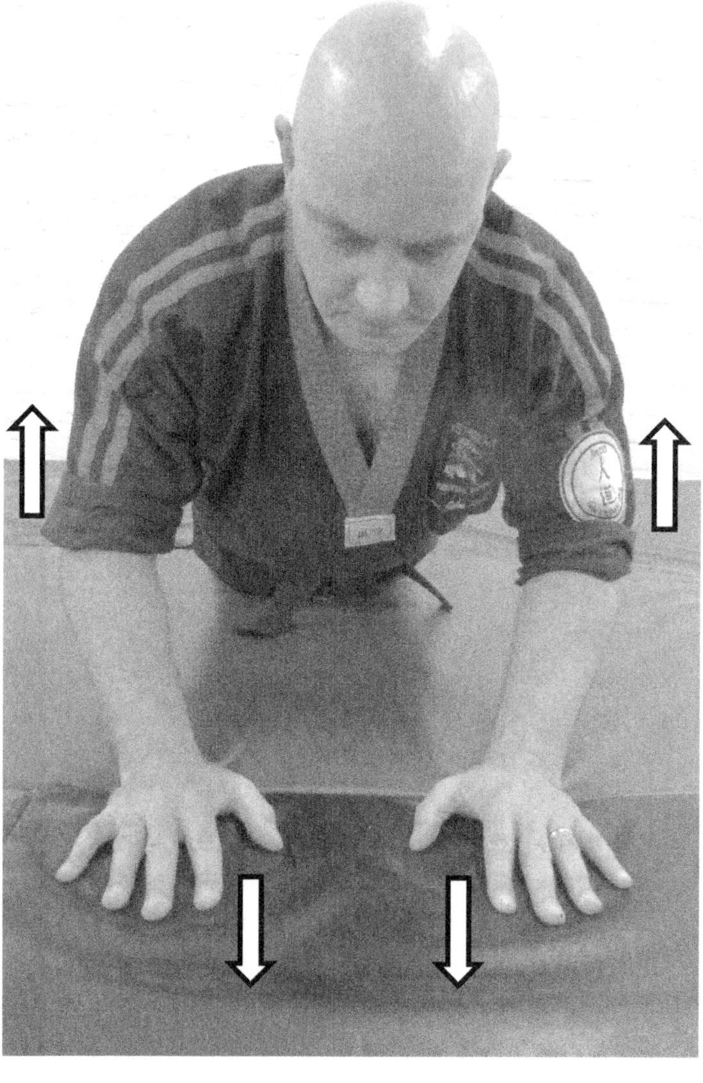

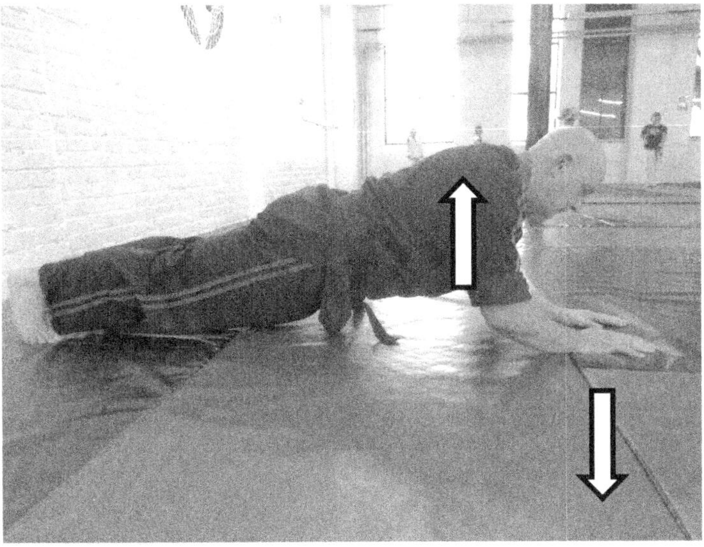

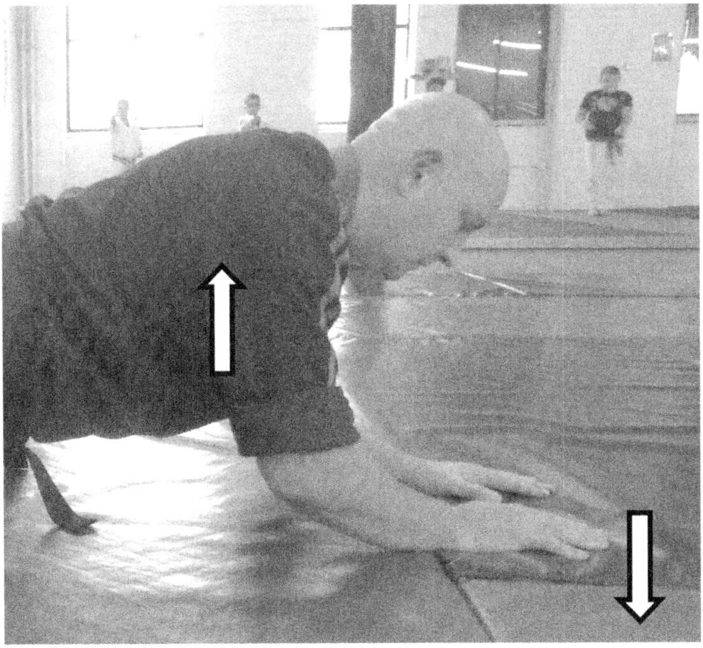

Arms – Triceps Over-Shoulder Belt Push-Down

Stand upright and hold an unfurled martial arts belt diagonally across your shoulder and back. One end should be at waist/hip height where it can be looped around one hand to secure it in position. The other end that is over your shoulder is looped around the hand performing the pushdown. Keep your elbow and arm close to your body, hold the belt firmly and perform a pushdown in as near to vertical action as you can manage. The belt should be long enough so that when your arm is approximately at the midpoint position, the isometric exercise can begin. Be sure to exercise both sides of the body by changing sides etc. The harder you engage the muscles, the more intense the exercise becomes, so always be sure to exercise at an intensity that best suits your current ability. When you perform an isometric exercise never hold your breath. Always breathe deeply and naturally, which will be about 10 full breaths in and out at a rate of about 1 second per full breath. Perform each exercise for no less than 7 seconds, and no longer than 10.

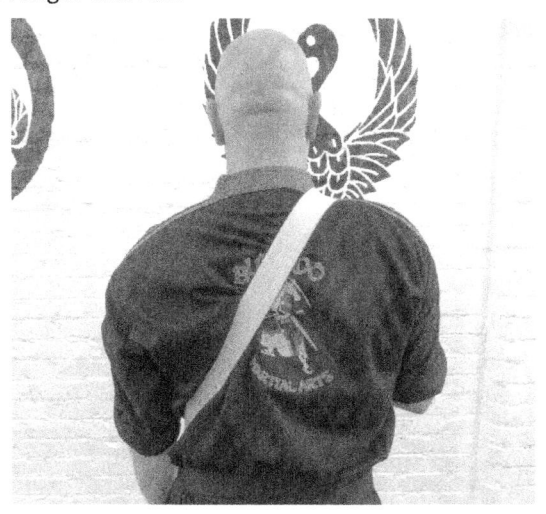

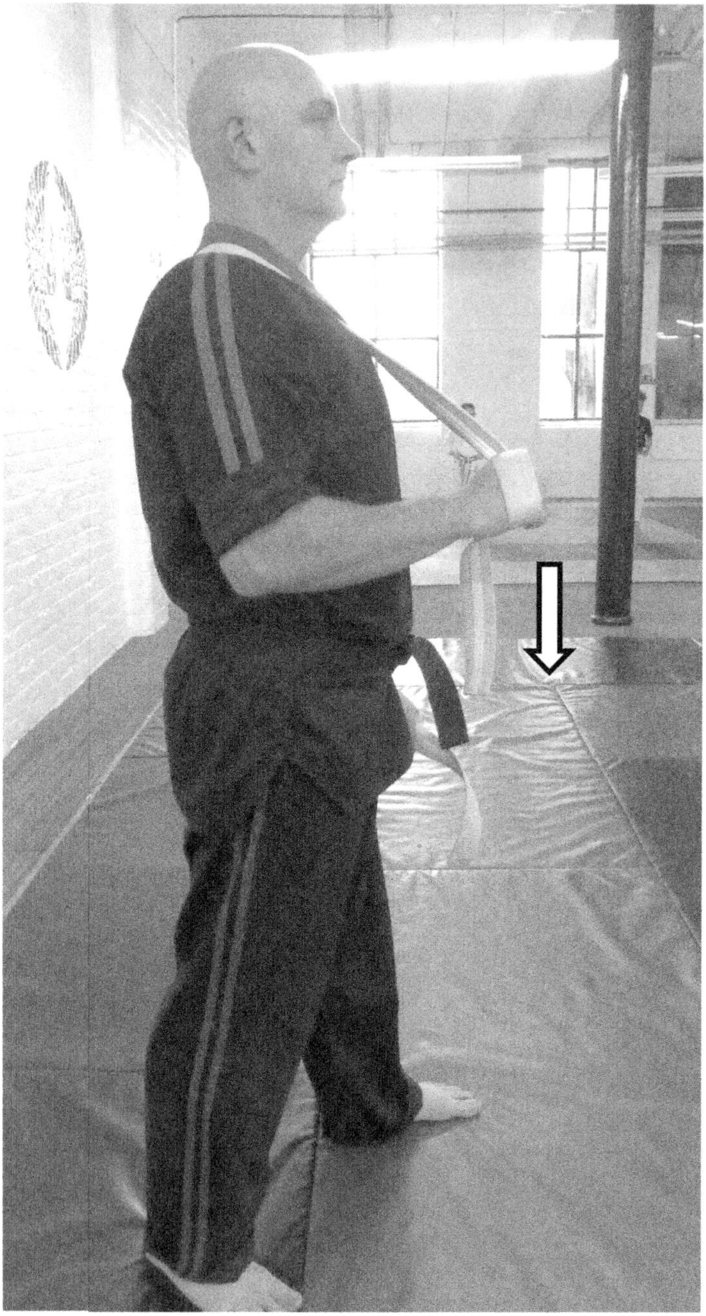

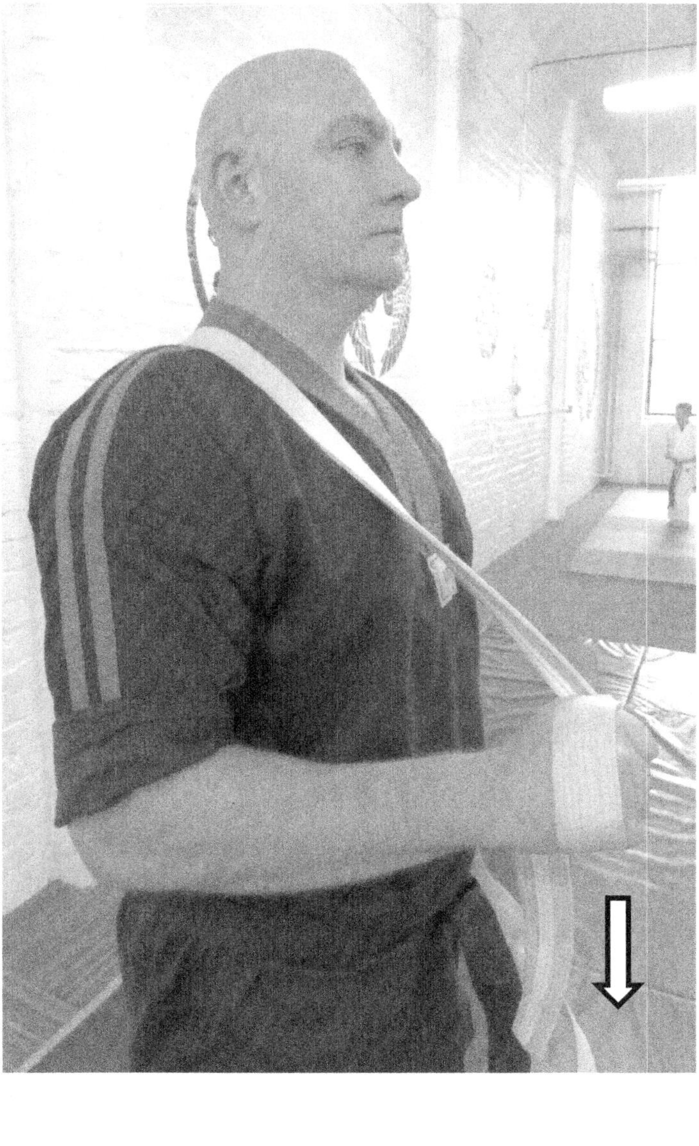

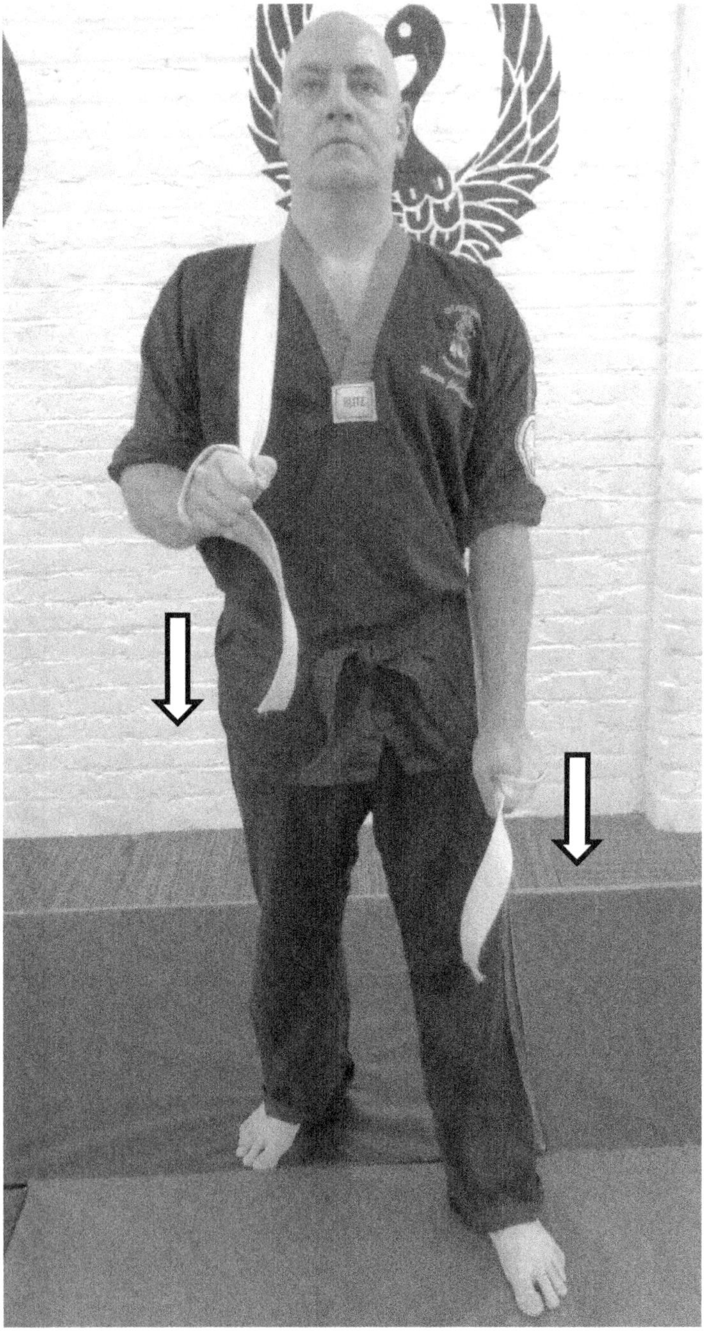

Arms – Triceps Over-Shoulder Belt Forward Push

Stand upright and hold an unfurled martial arts belt diagonally across your shoulder and back. One end should be at waist/hip height where it can be looped around one hand to secure it in position. The other end that is over your shoulder is looped around the hand performing the forward push. Lift your arm to be exercised so that the lower upper part is approximately horizontal to the floor, and so that your forearm is held vertically. The belt should be long enough so that when your arm is approximately at the midpoint position extended forwards, the isometric exercise can begin. Be sure to exercise both sides of the body by changing sides etc. The harder you engage the muscles, the more intense the exercise becomes, so always be sure to exercise at an intensity that best suits your current ability. When you perform an isometric exercise never hold your breath. Always breathe deeply and naturally, which will be about 10 full breaths in and out at a rate of about 1 second per full breath. Perform each exercise for no less than 7 seconds, and no longer than 10.

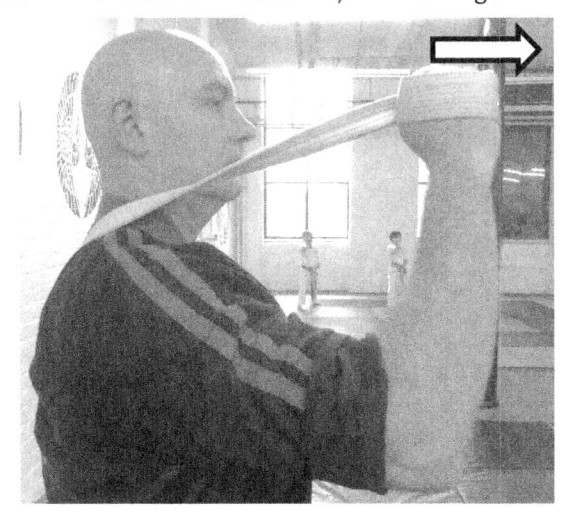

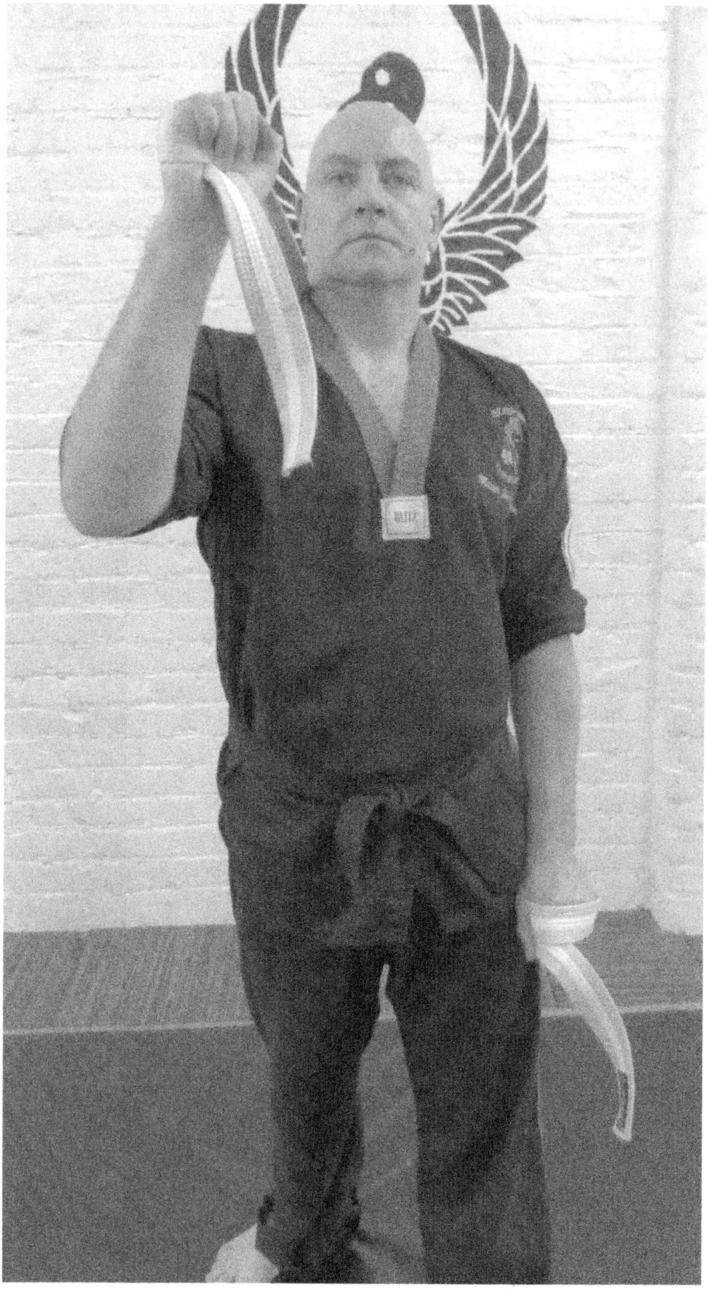

146

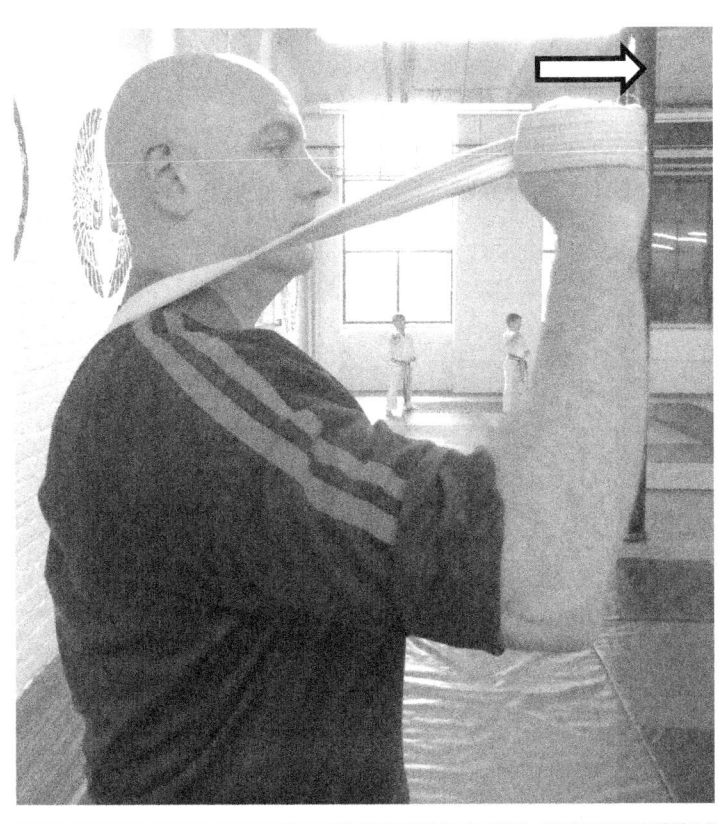

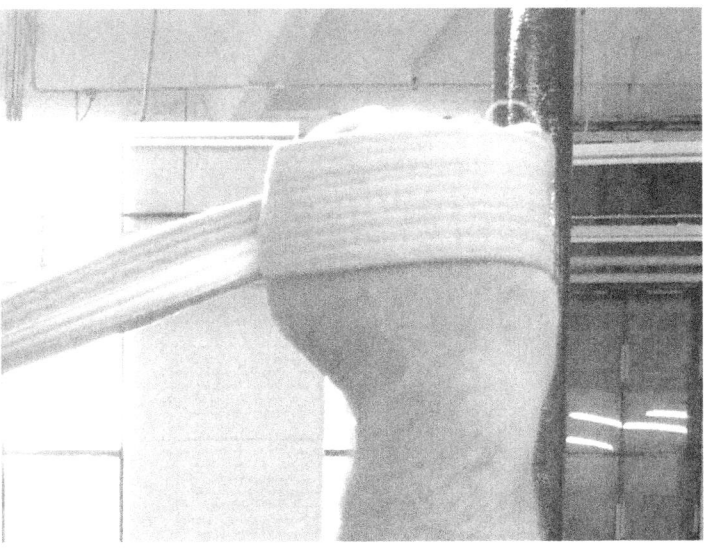

Arms – Triceps Overhead Press

Stand upright and hold an unfurled martial arts belt wrapped around your hand and held directly overhead at arm's length. The other end should fall down your back to be gripped and secured by the other hand at approximately waist/hip height. The arm held overhead should be bent at the elbow at approximately 90 degrees/midpoint. At the same time, the upper part of the arm should remain as vertical as possible with the elbow tip pointing to the ceiling. Apply force as if to try and extend the upper hand and forearm upwards, this will be thwarted by the length of the belt secured by the other hand at waist height. The isometric exercise can then begin. The harder you engage the muscles, the more intense the exercise becomes, so always be sure to exercise at an intensity that best suits your current ability. When you perform an isometric exercise never hold your breath. Always breathe deeply and naturally, which will be about 10 full breaths in and out at a rate of about 1 second per full breath. Perform each exercise for no less than 7 seconds, and no longer than 10. Be sure to exercise both sides of the body.

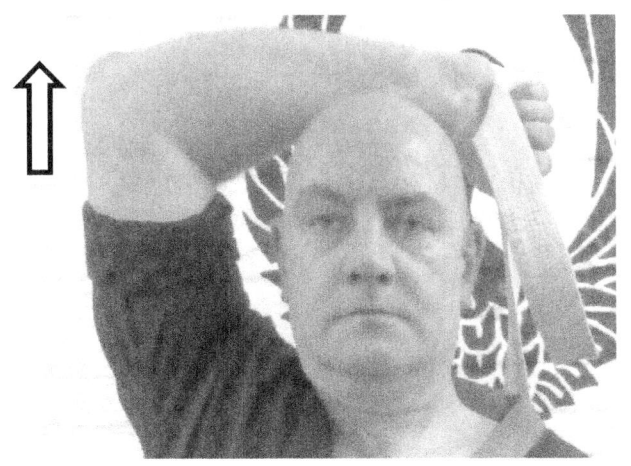

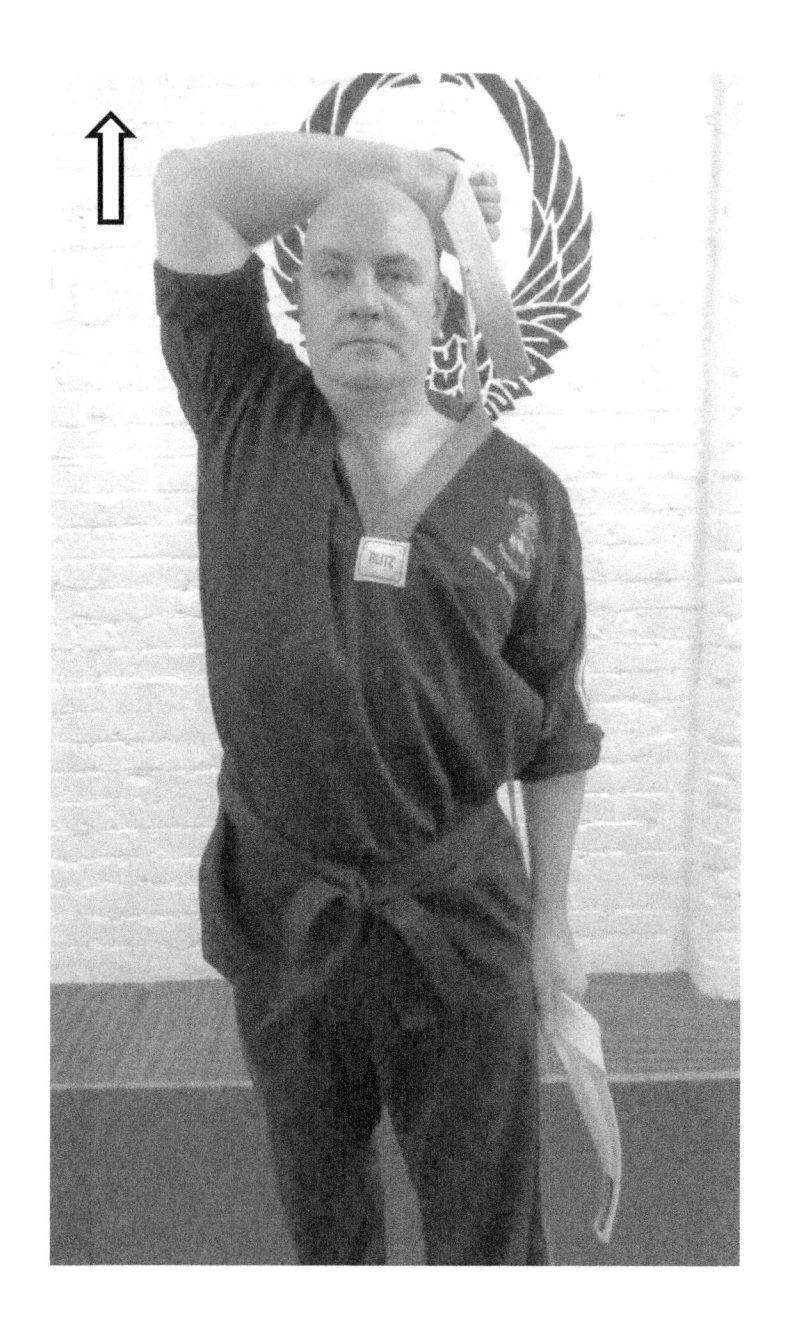

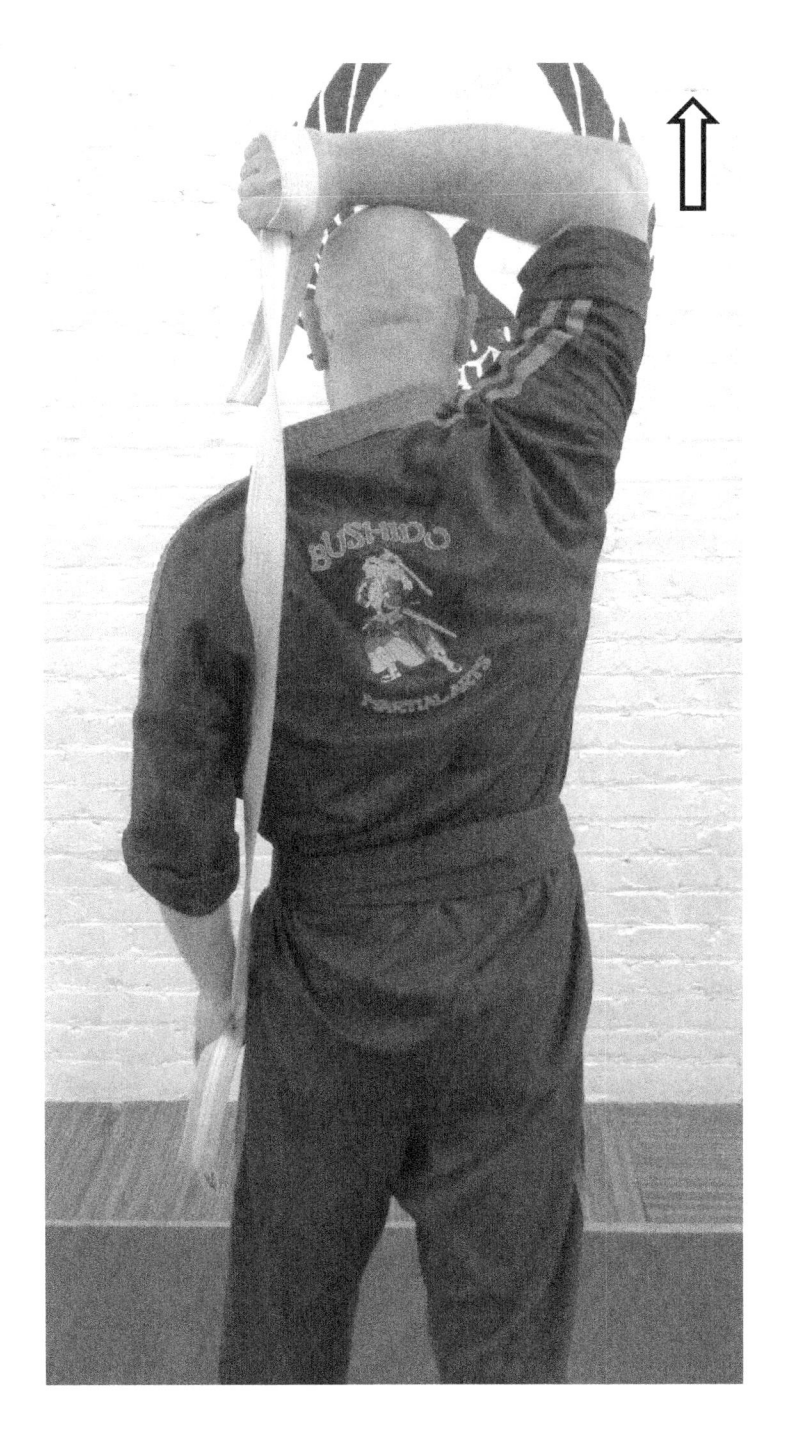

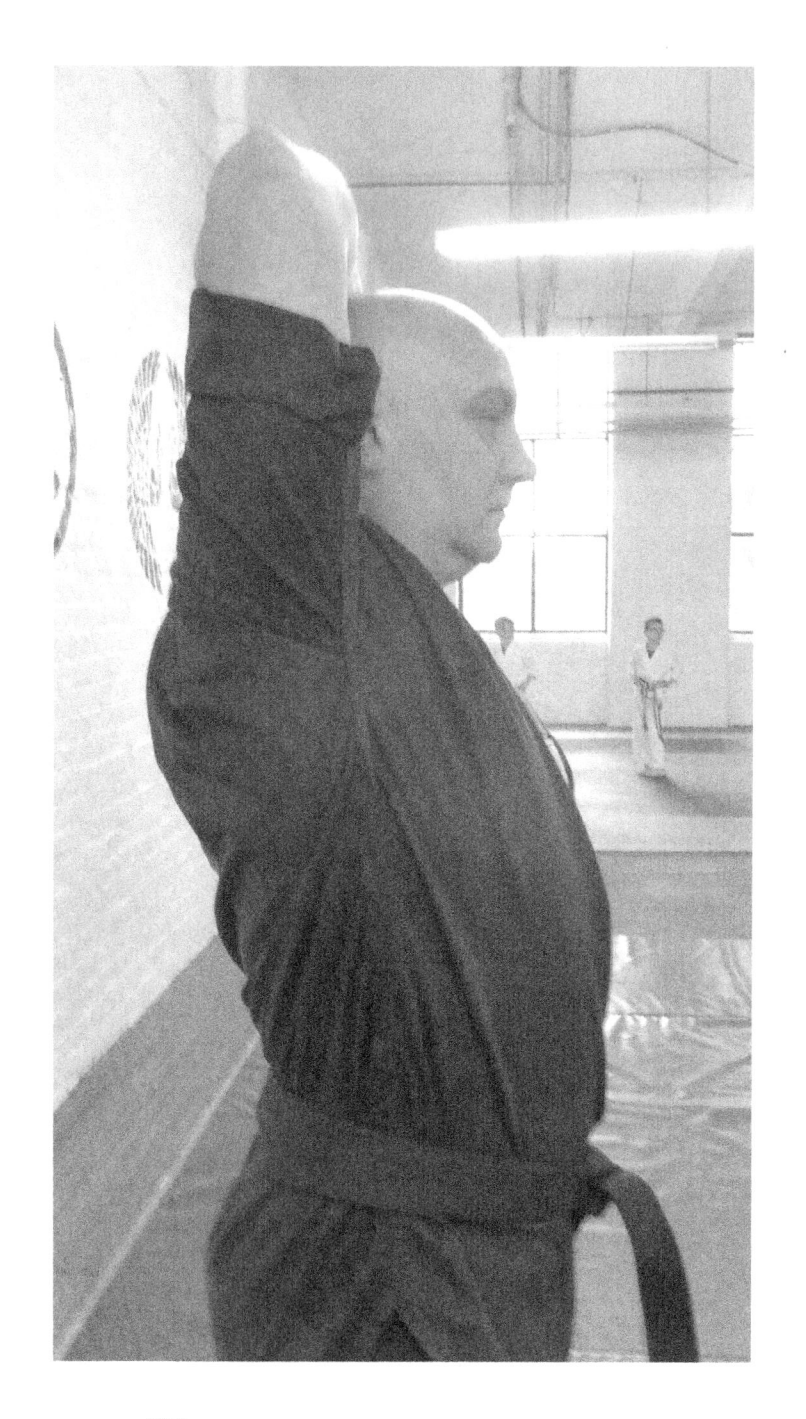

Lower Back–Belt Deadlift

Stand on an evenly laid out martial arts belt with your feet approximately shoulder-width apart. Bend into a semi-squat position with the knees bent and the back straight, bending forward only at the hips. Take hold of each one, one in each hand and loop the belt around the hands. In this position, use the lower back, buttocks, and upper thighs as the driving muscles as you attempt to lift the belt evenly. Naturally, you will not be able to do this as the belt is secured by your feet. An isometric exercise may be performed at any point according to how long the end sections of the belt are allowed to be. When you have assumed your ideal deadlift position, then perform the isometric exercise. The harder you engage the muscles, the more intense the exercise becomes, so always be sure to exercise at an intensity that best suits your current ability. When you perform an isometric exercise never hold your breath. Always breathe deeply and naturally, which will be about 10 full breaths in and out at a rate of about 1 second per full breath. Perform each exercise for no less than 7 seconds, and no longer than 10.

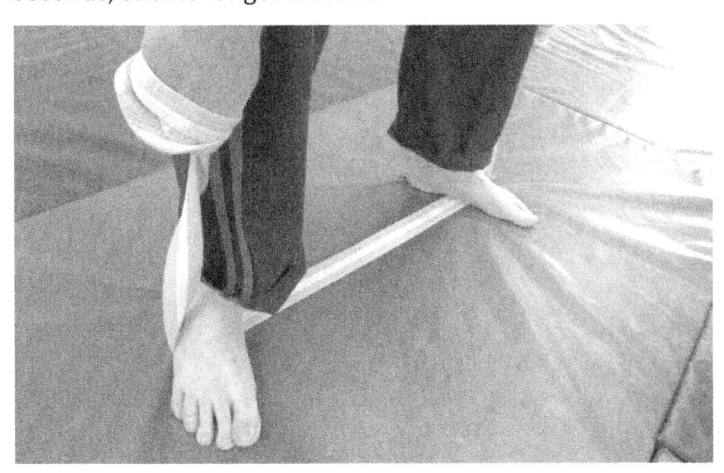

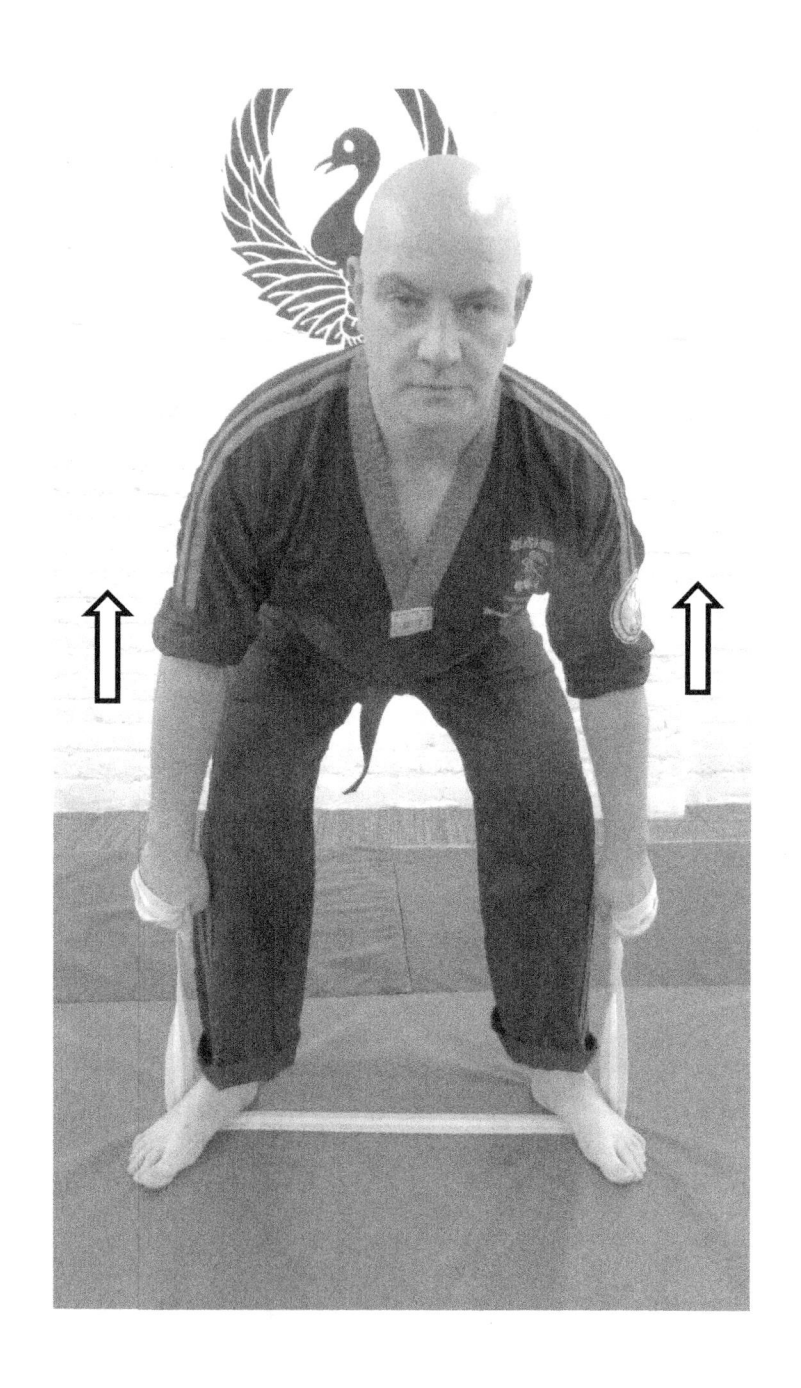

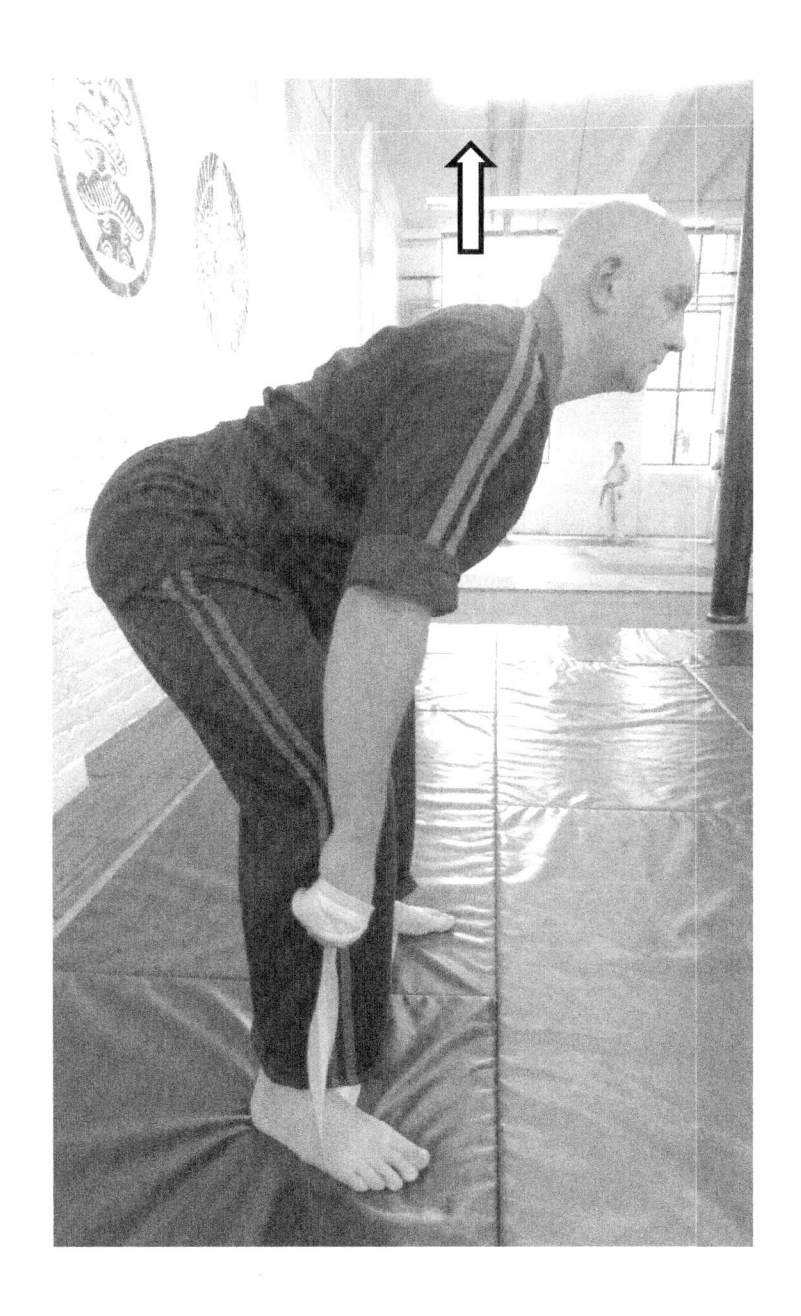

Lower Back – Good Morning Bend with Belt

Stand with your feet approximately shoulder-width apart. Bend the knees slightly and keep them in a locked-bent position. As you bend forward, make sure that you keep your back straight and bend only from the hip. Bend forward to a low point where the torso is as near as possible to horizontal. In this position, extend both arms forward at approximately shoulder-width apart and hold a martial arts belt between them, pulling it apart slightly as you do so. When you have assumed your ideal good morning position, hold it, and then perform the isometric exercise.

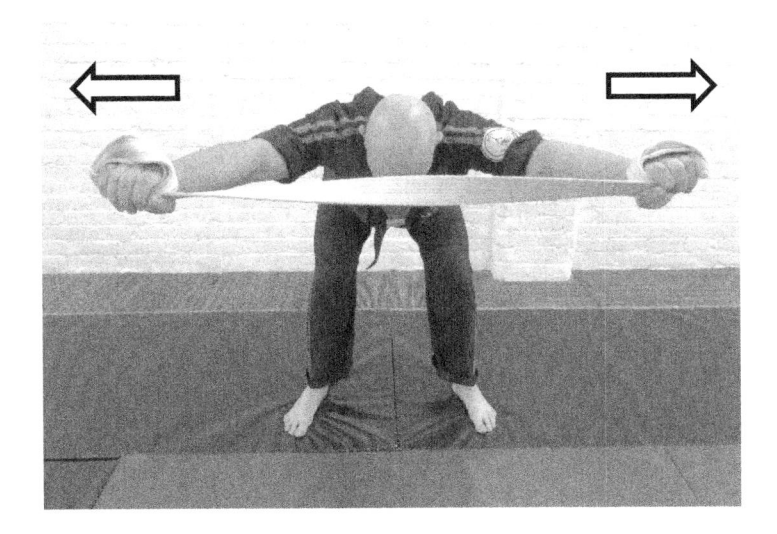

The harder you engage the muscles, the more intense the exercise becomes, so always be sure to exercise at an intensity that best suits your current ability. When you perform an isometric exercise never hold your breath. Always breathe deeply and naturally, which will be about 10 full breaths in and out at a rate of about 1 second per full breath. Perform each exercise for no less than 7 seconds, and no longer than 10.

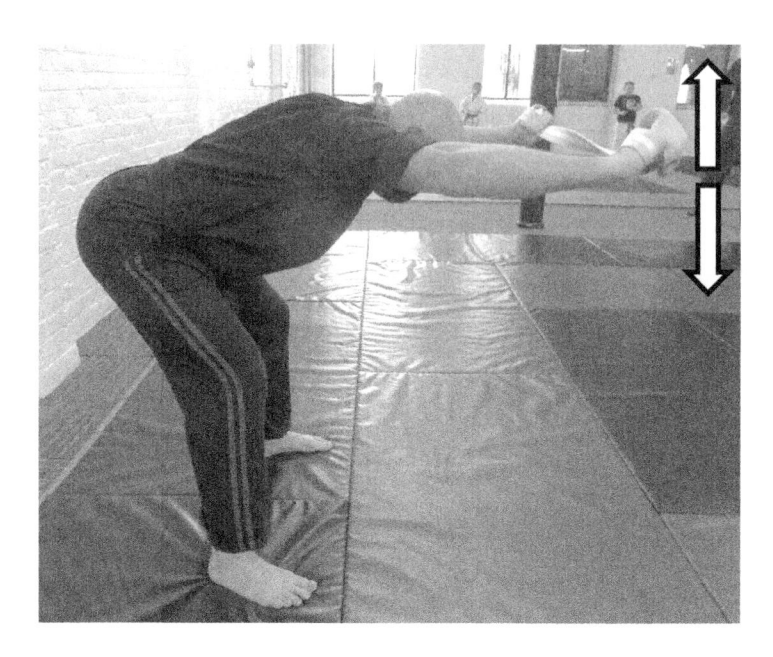

Lower Back – Variation – Kneeling Good Morning

Kneel on your haunches with your legs approximately shoulder-width apart. As you bend forward, make sure that you keep your back straight and bend only from the hip. Bend forward to a low point where the torso is as near as possible to horizontal. When you have assumed your ideal kneeling good morning position, then hold it and perform the isometric exercise.

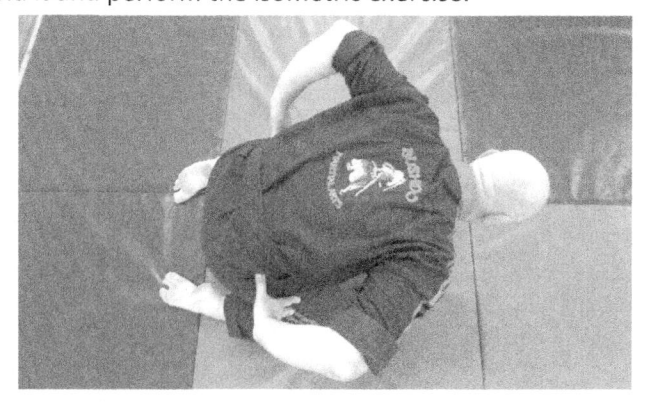

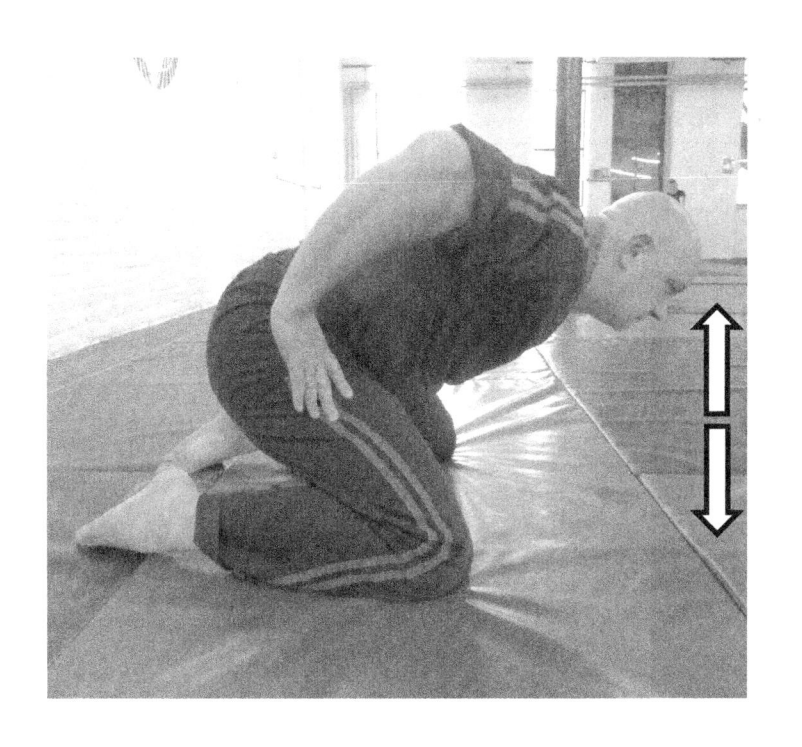

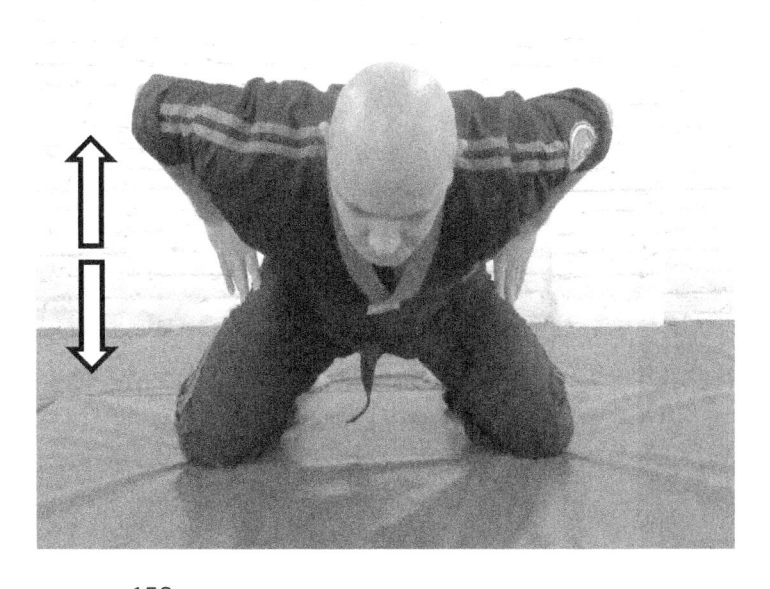

Lower Back – Variation
Kneeling Good Morning Arms Extended

Kneel on your haunches with your legs approximately shoulder-width apart. As you bend forward, make sure that you keep your back straight and bend only from the hip. Bend forward to a low point where the torso is as near as possible to horizontal. Extend your hands and arms as far forward as possible. Aim to eventually assume a position with the arms fully extended, and if you cannot do this right away, then work up to it gradually. When you have assumed your ideal kneeling good morning position with your arms extended, hold it, and perform the standard isometric exercise for between 7 and 10 seconds.

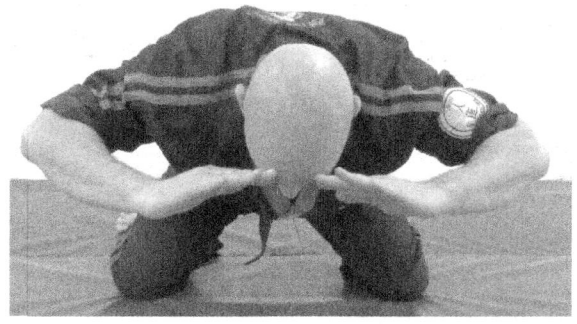

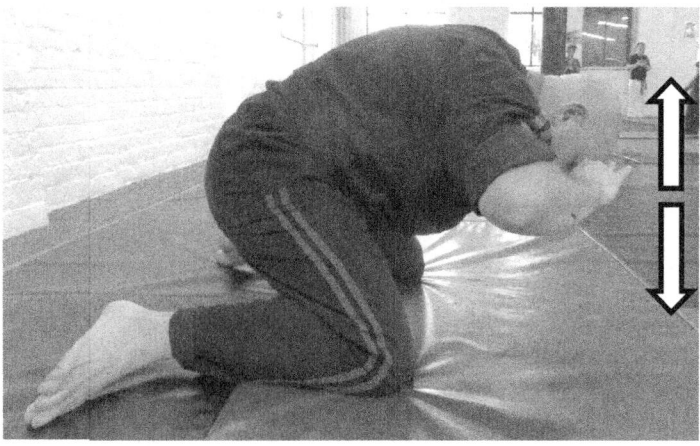

Lower Back – Superhero

Lie flat on the floor face down. Extend your hands and arms as far forward as possible. Aim to eventually assume a position with the arms fully extended, and if you cannot do this right away, then work up to it gradually. In this position, simultaneously raise both your extended arms and shoulders together with your legs. When you have assumed your ideal superhero position with your arms extended, hold it, and perform the isometric exercise.

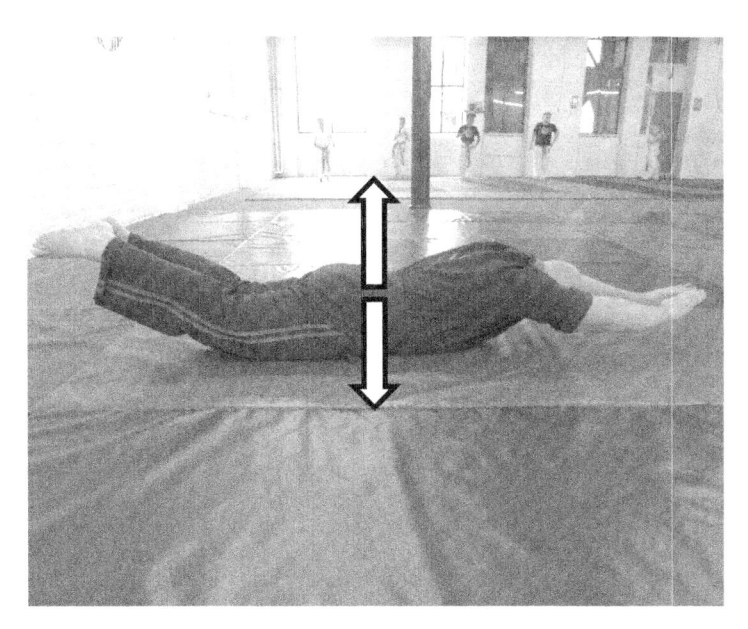

The harder you engage the muscles, the more intense the exercise becomes, so always be sure to exercise at an intensity that best suits your current ability. When you perform an isometric exercise never hold your breath. Always breathe deeply and naturally, which will be about 10 full breaths in and out at a rate of about 1 second per full breath. Perform each exercise for no less than 7 seconds, and no longer than 10.

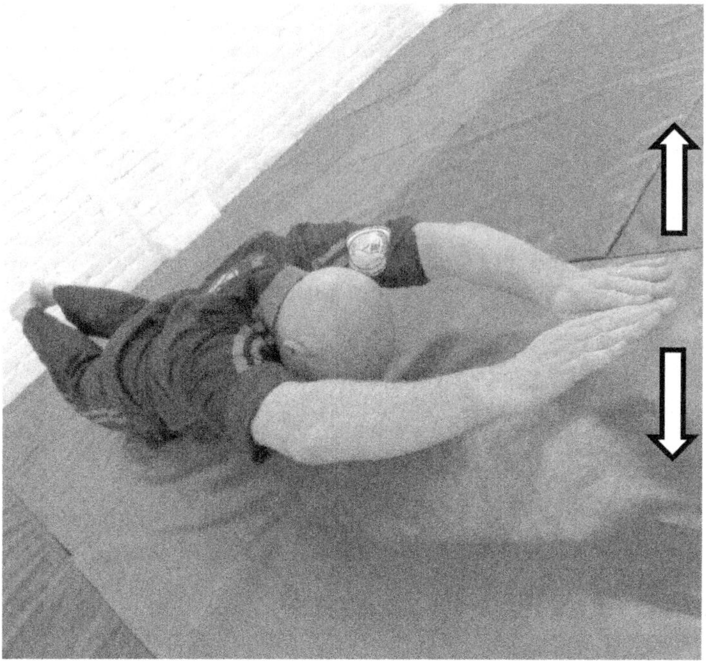

Upper Back – Chest Level Belt Pull-Apart

Stand upright with your feet approximately shoulder-width apart. Hold an unfurled martial arts belt at chest level. Keep your hands close together and with the ends of the belt wrapped around the hands. Keep your arms and elbows also up at chest level so they are horizontal to the floor. In this position, engage the muscles of the upper back as you attempt to pull the belt apart. When you have assumed your ideal position, hold it, and perform the isometric exercise.

The harder you engage the muscles, the more intense the exercise becomes, so always be sure to exercise at an intensity that best suits your current ability. When you perform an isometric exercise never hold your breath. Always breathe deeply and naturally, which will be about 10 full breaths in and out at a rate of about 1 second per full breath. Perform each exercise for no less than 7 seconds, and no longer than 10.

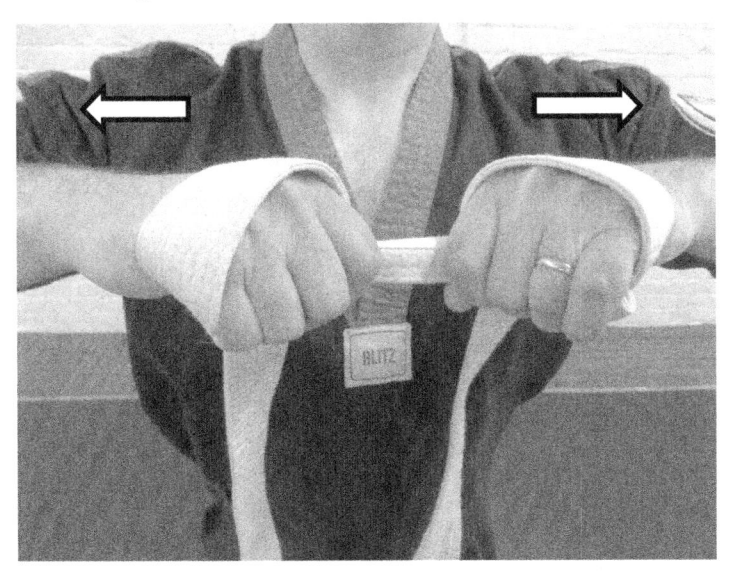

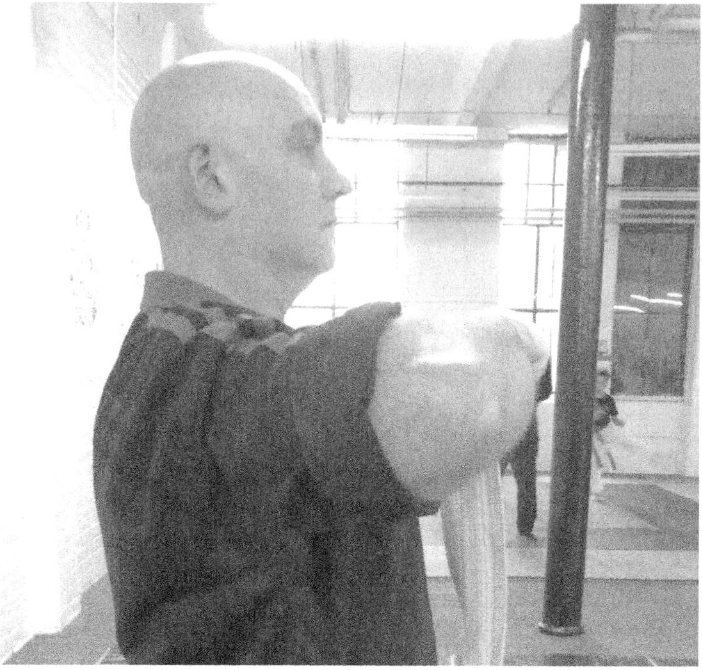

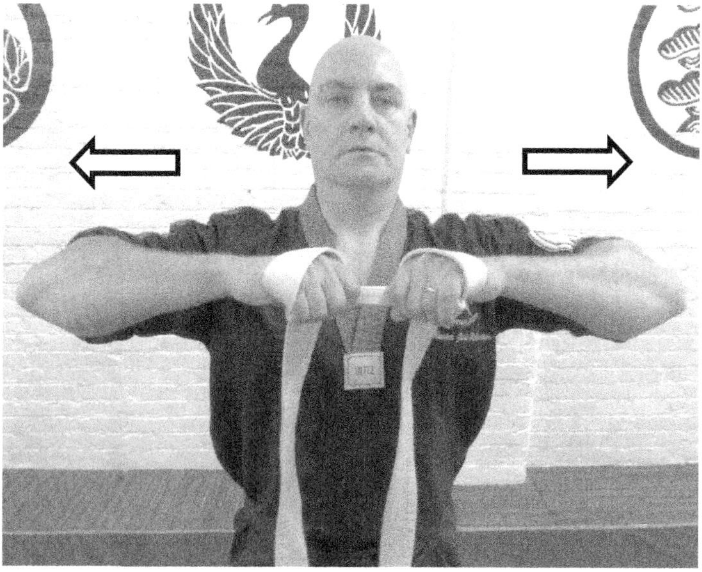

Upper Back –
Chest Level Pull-Apart Variation

If no belt is available, or if you simply do not wish to use one, then the same exercise can be performed by interlocking the hands as shown.

NOTE: Using a belt to perform this exercise has a distinct advantage. It allows multiple positions to be performed by varying the length of the belt allowed between the hands. However, both methods have merit and deliver excellent results. Perform the isometric exercise technique in the same way.

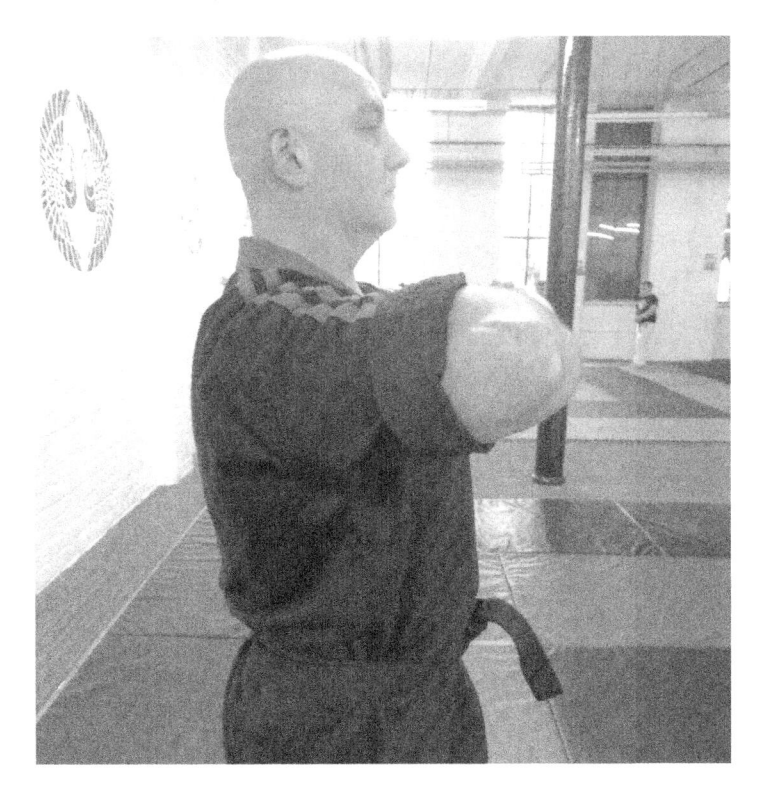

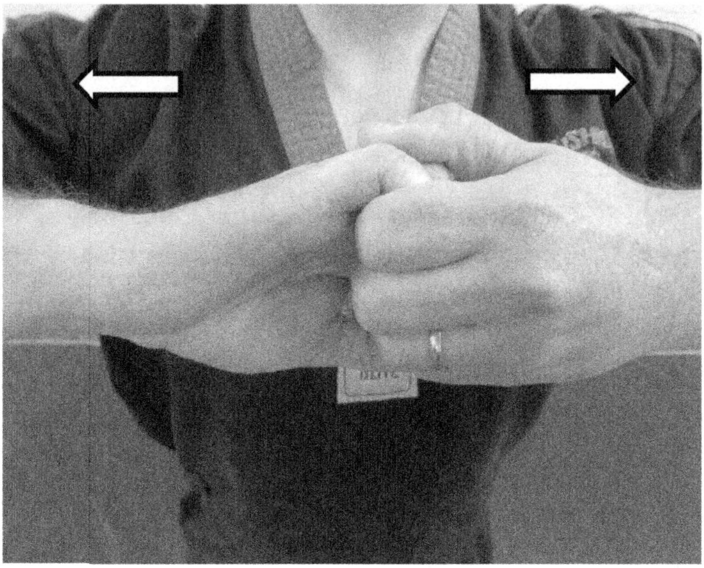

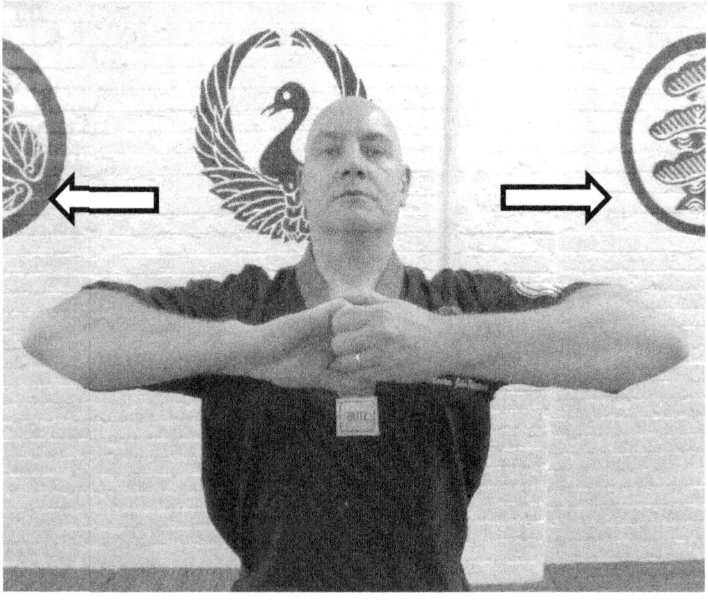

Upper Back – Overhead Belt Pull-Apart

Stand upright with your feet approximately shoulder-width apart. Hold an unfurled martial arts belt above your head with your arms held as vertically as possible. Keep your hands close together and with the ends of the belt wrapped around the hands. In this position, engage the muscles of the upper back as you attempt to pull the belt apart, simultaneously sideways and downwards. When you have assumed your ideal position, hold it, and perform the isometric exercise.

The harder you engage the muscles, the more intense the exercise becomes, so always be sure to exercise at an intensity that best suits your current ability. When you perform an isometric exercise never hold your breath. Always breathe deeply and naturally, which will be about 10 full breaths in and out at a rate of about 1 second per full breath. Perform each exercise for no less than 7 seconds, and no longer than 10.

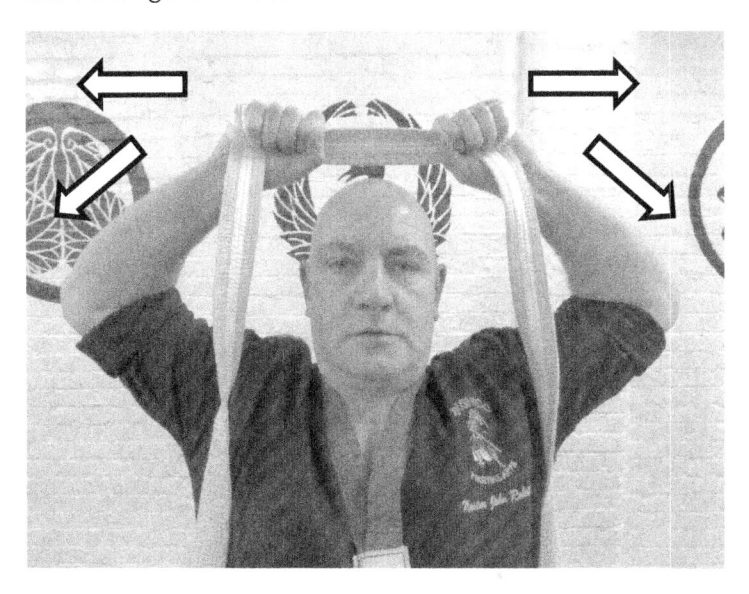

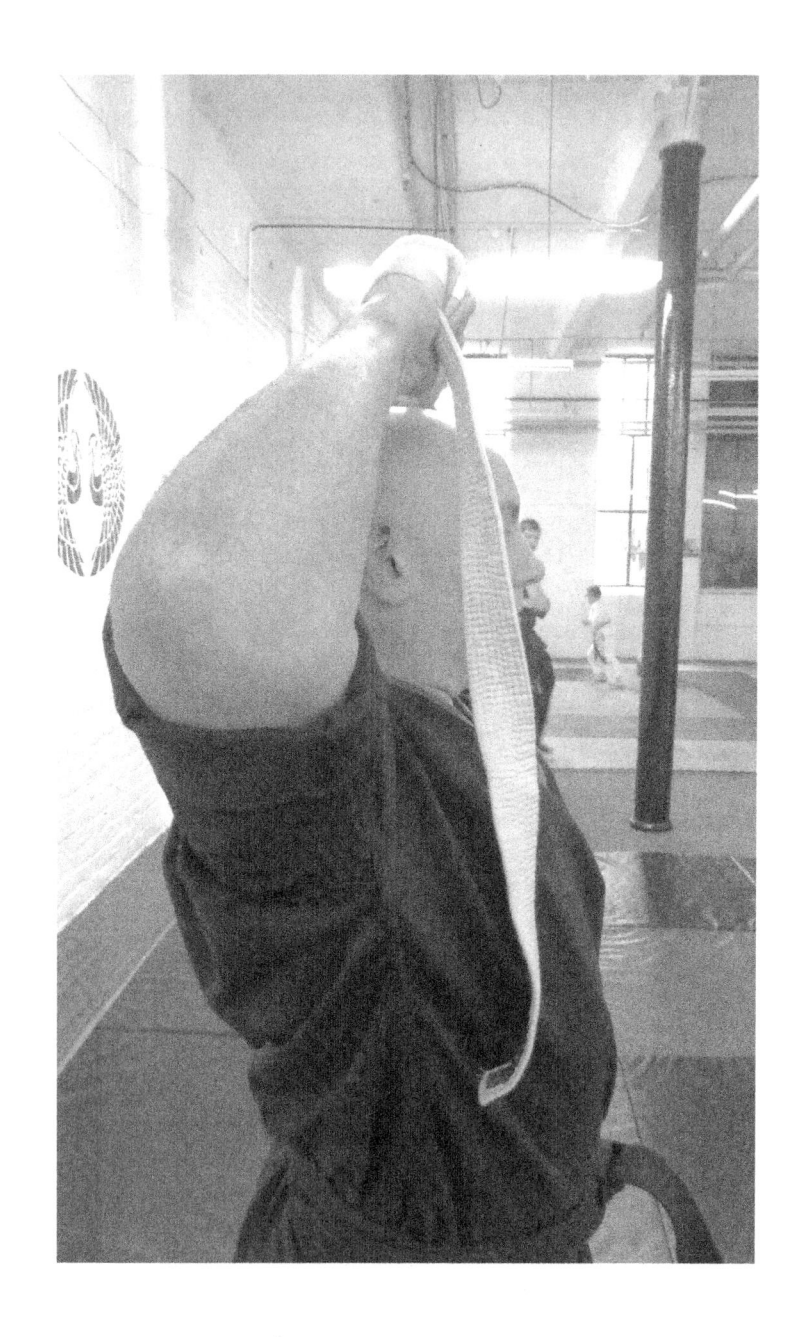

Upper Back – Overhead Pull-Apart Variation

If no belt is available, or if you simply do not wish to use one, then the same exercise can be performed by interlocking the hands as shown.

NOTE: Using a belt to perform this exercise has a distinct advantage. It allows multiple positions to be performed by varying the length of the belt allowed between the hands.

However, both methods have merit and deliver excellent results. Perform the isometric exercise technique in the same way.

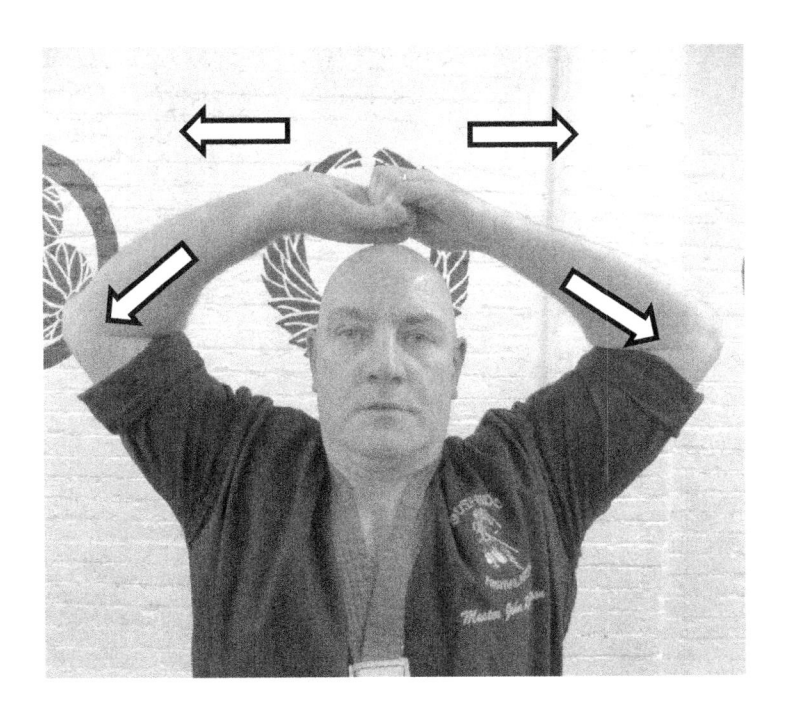

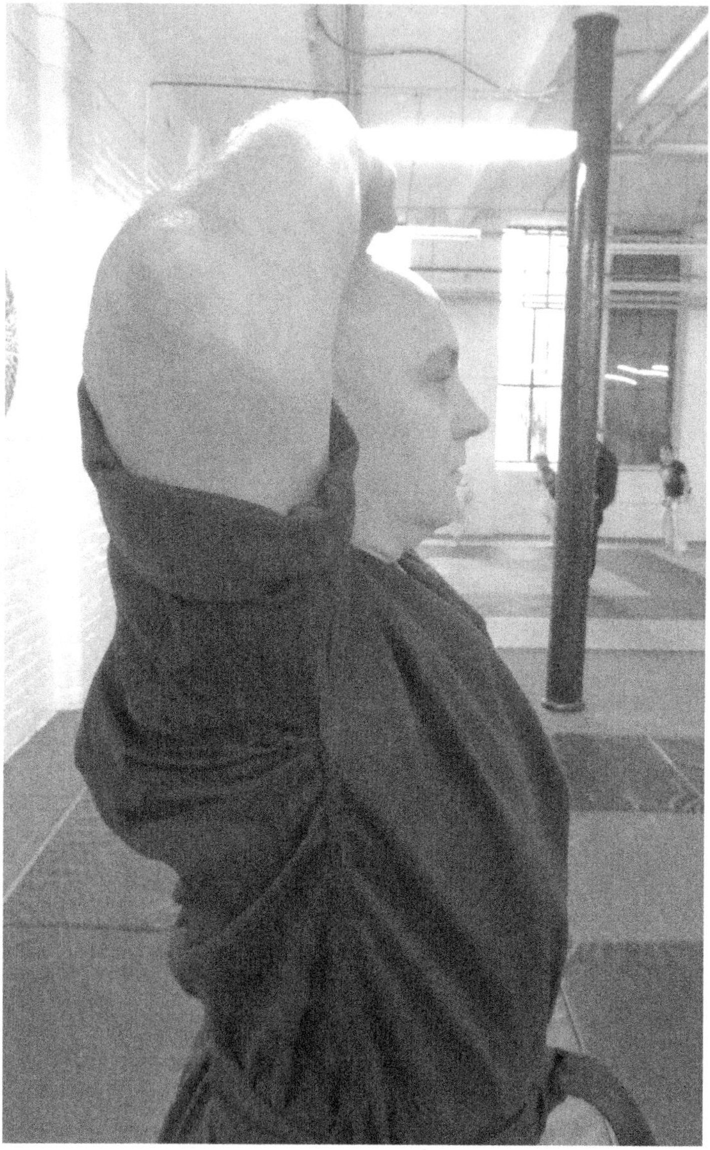

Upper Back – Seated Belt Knee Row

Sit on a chair, bench, or any solid object. Raise one leg and wrap an unfurled martial arts belt evenly around the upper shin close to the knee. Hold each end of the belt, one in each hand.

Wrap the belt around the hands to leave a sufficient length of the belt so that when the arms are pulled backwards, the knee bracing the belt prevents the arms from moving too far. Aim to perform the exercise with an approximately 90-degree bend of the elbows at the midpoint.

When you pull back with the arms, leading with the elbows, be sure to keep the arms close to the body and not to let the elbows creep out sideways during the exercise. In this position, engage the muscles of the upper back as you attempt to pull the knee back.

The knee and thigh can offset this pull by pushing against it to generate the required exercise resistance. When you have assumed your ideal position, hold it, and perform the isometric exercise.

The harder you engage the muscles, the more intense the exercise becomes, so always be sure to exercise at an intensity that best suits your current ability.

When you perform an isometric exercise never hold your breath. Always breathe deeply and naturally, which will be about 10 full breaths in and out at a rate of about 1 second

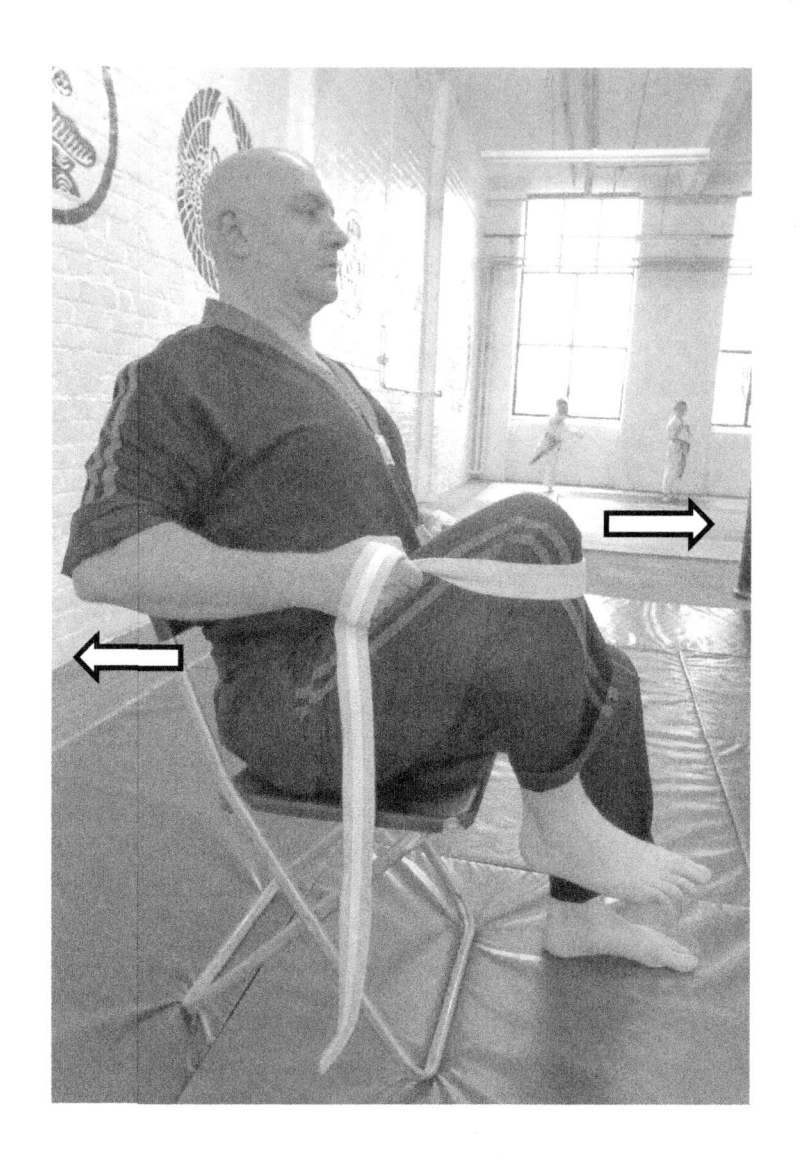

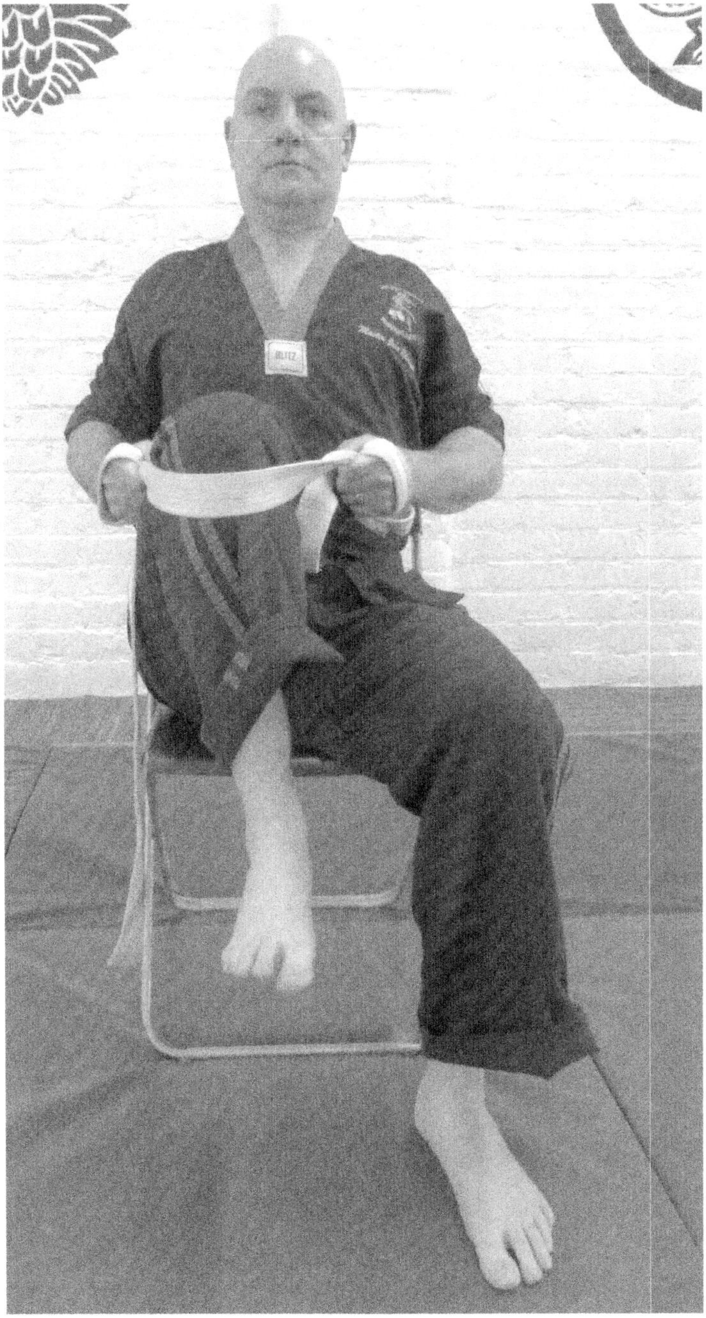

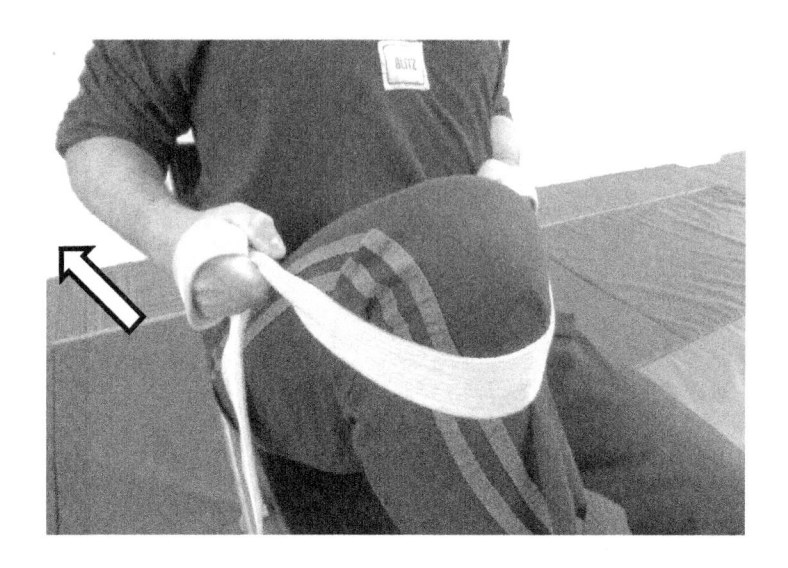

Upper Back – Seated Knee Row Variation

A variation to the seated belt knee row is to perform the exercise without a belt. This is done by clasping the hands together and interlocking fingers as needed over the knee and upper shin. Perform the isometric exercise in the same way.

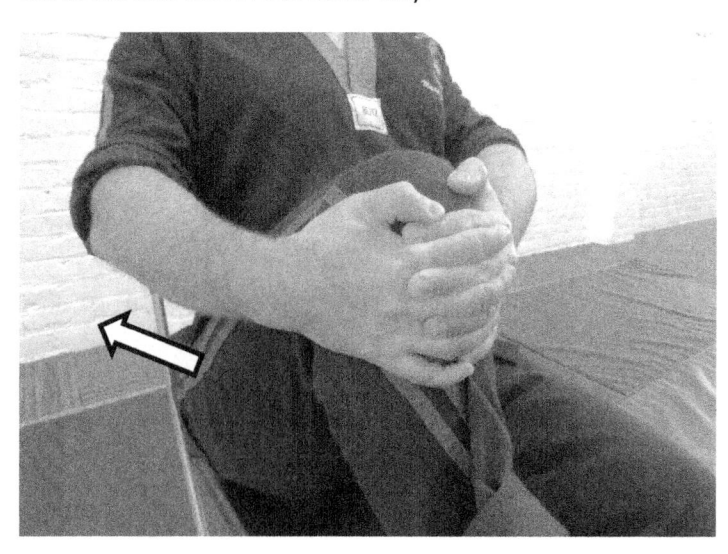

174

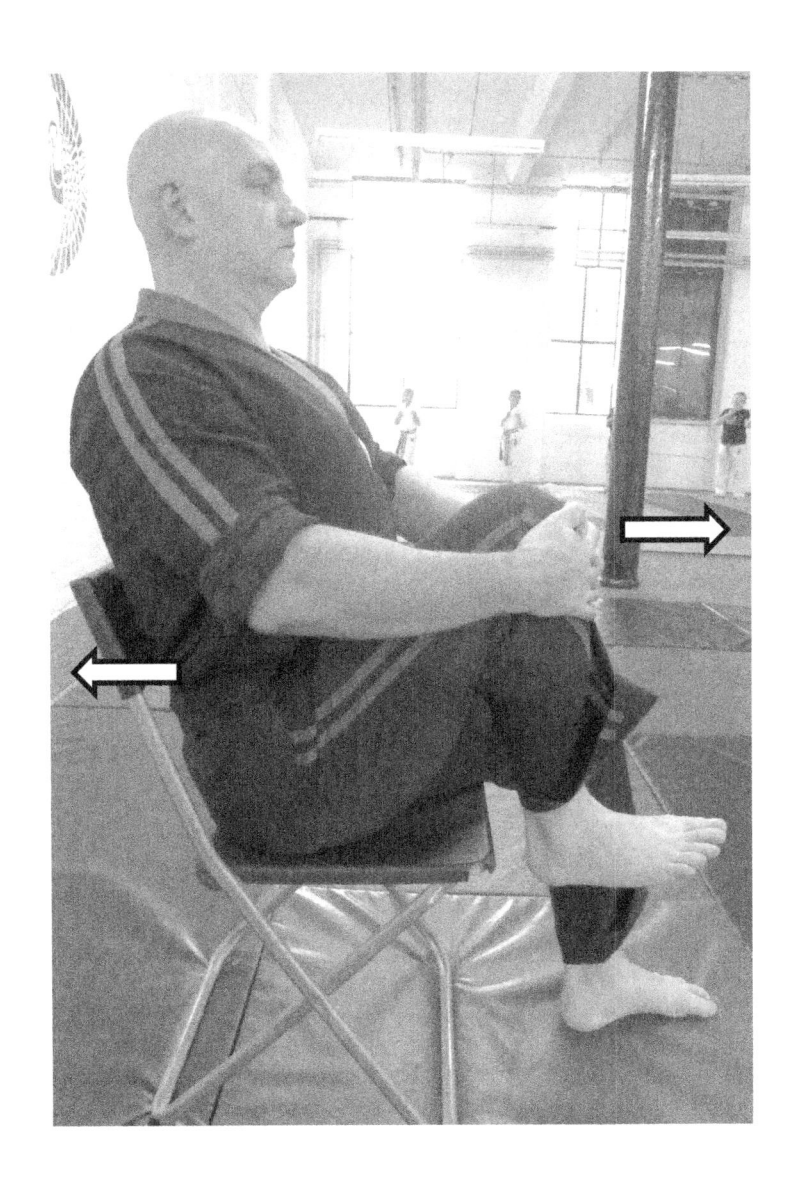

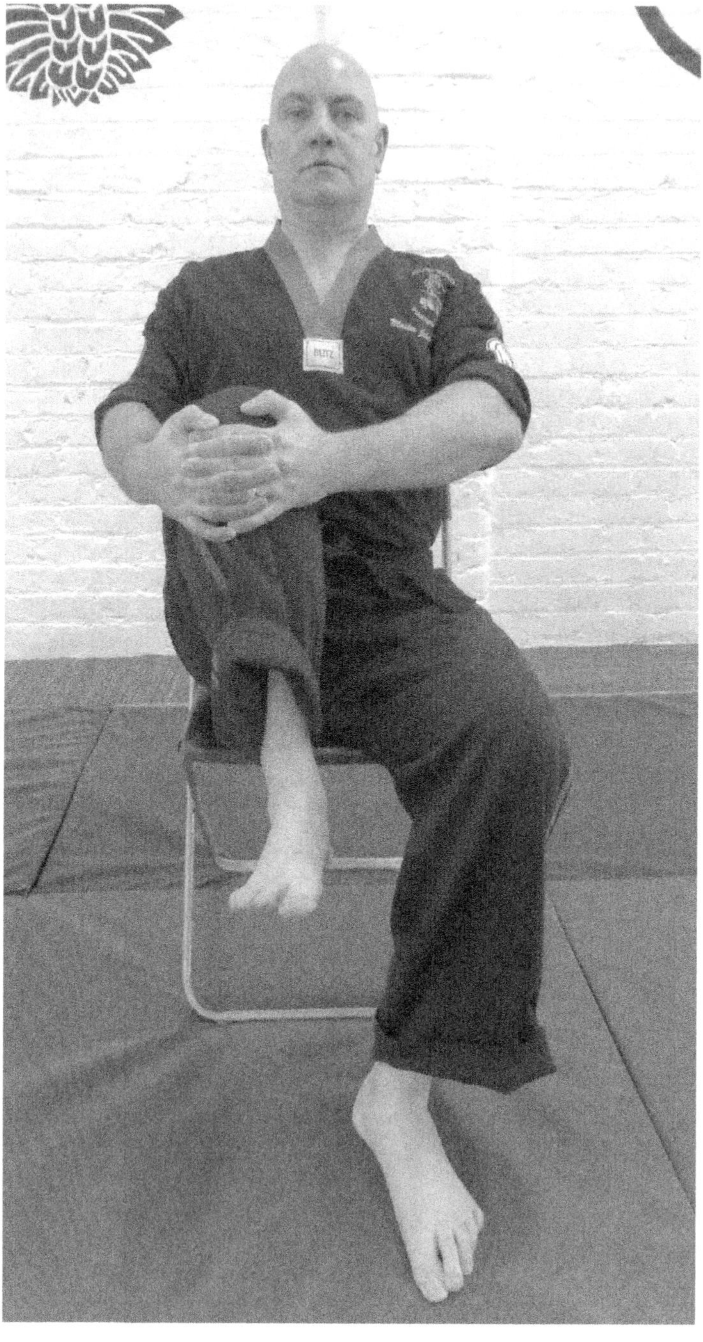

Upper Back – Seated Belt Knee Row Floor

Sit on the mat or the floor with your torso upright and both legs extended. Bend both legs slightly and lock them in that position. Place an unfurled martial arts belt, or similar, securely around both feet. Hold each end of the belt, one in each hand.

Wrap the belt around the hands to leave a sufficient length of the belt so that when the arms are pulled backwards, the feet bracing the belt prevent the arms from moving too far. Aim to perform the exercise with an approximately 90-degree bend of the elbows at the midpoint.

When you pull back with the arms, leading with the elbows, be sure to keep the arms close to the body and not to let the elbows creep out sideways during the exercise. In this position, engage the muscles of the upper back as you attempt to pull the feet back.

The feet and legs can easily offset this pull by pushing against the belt to generate the required exercise resistance. When you have assumed your ideal position, hold it, and perform the isometric exercise.

The harder you engage the muscles, the more intense the exercise becomes, so always be sure to exercise at an intensity that best suits your current ability.

When you perform an isometric exercise never hold your breath. Always breathe deeply and naturally, which will be about 10 full breaths in and out at a rate of about 1 second per full breath. Perform each exercise for no less than 7 seconds, and no longer than 10.

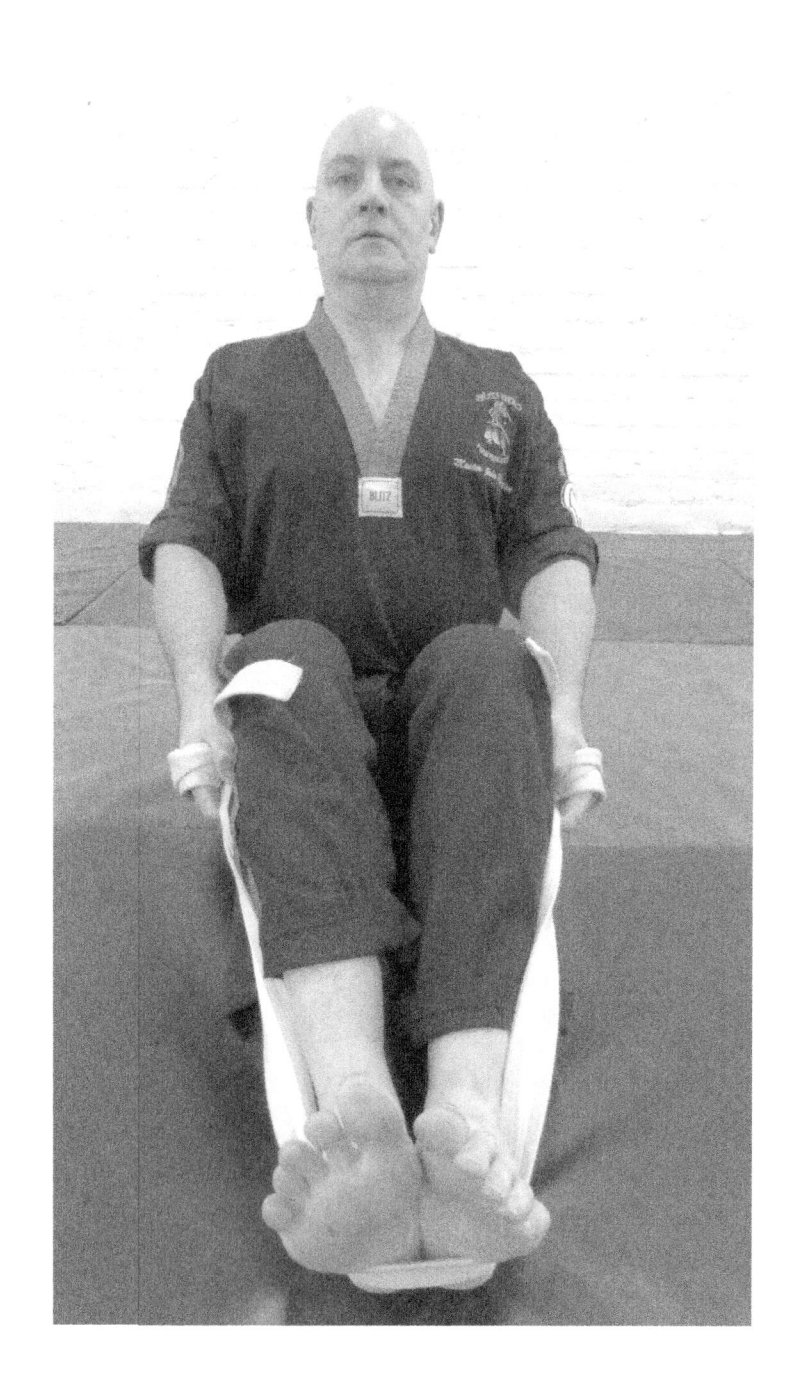

178

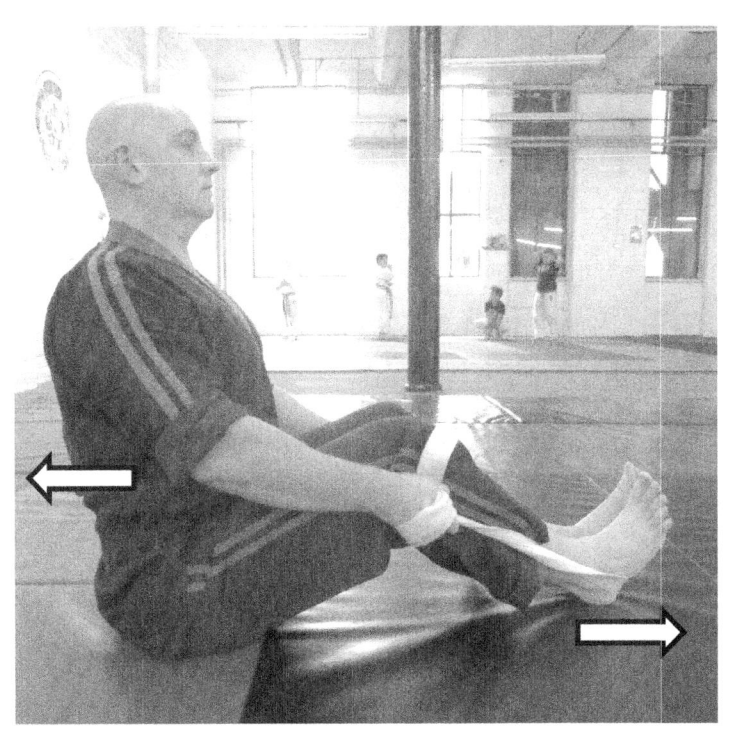

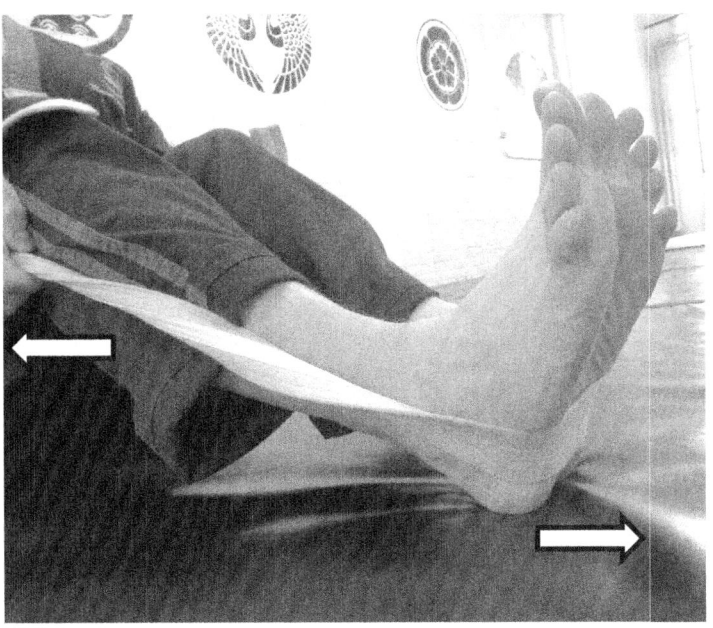

Upper Back – Standing Single Arm Belt Row

Stand upright in a forward stance. It does not matter if it is a left or right stance as you will exercise both sides of the body when one exercise is completed by changing to the other leg etc. Hold an unfurled martial arts belt, or similar, in both hands and with it looped under the leading foot. Start with the torso facing forward, and pull the arm and elbow back in a rowing action on the side holding the *slightly* longer section of the belt.

Make sure that the belt is only long enough to stop you so that your arm is at approximately 90 degrees at the midpoint. Use the muscles of the upper back to generate the force of the pull and brace your torso by using the other arm on the forward thigh while it secures the other end of the belt.

fully twisting to the side and back so that you are at about the halfway position when you perform the exercise. Use the oblique abdominal muscles and the muscles of the hip and lower back to drive the exercise. When you have assumed your ideal position, hold it, and perform the isometric exercise.

The harder you engage the muscles, the more intense the exercise becomes, so always be sure to exercise at an intensity that best suits your current ability. When you perform an isometric exercise never hold your breath.

Always breathe deeply and naturally, which will be about 10 full breaths in and out at a rate of about 1 second per full breath. Perform each exercise for no less than 7 seconds, and no longer than 10. Be sure to exercise both sides of the body by changing sides etc.

181

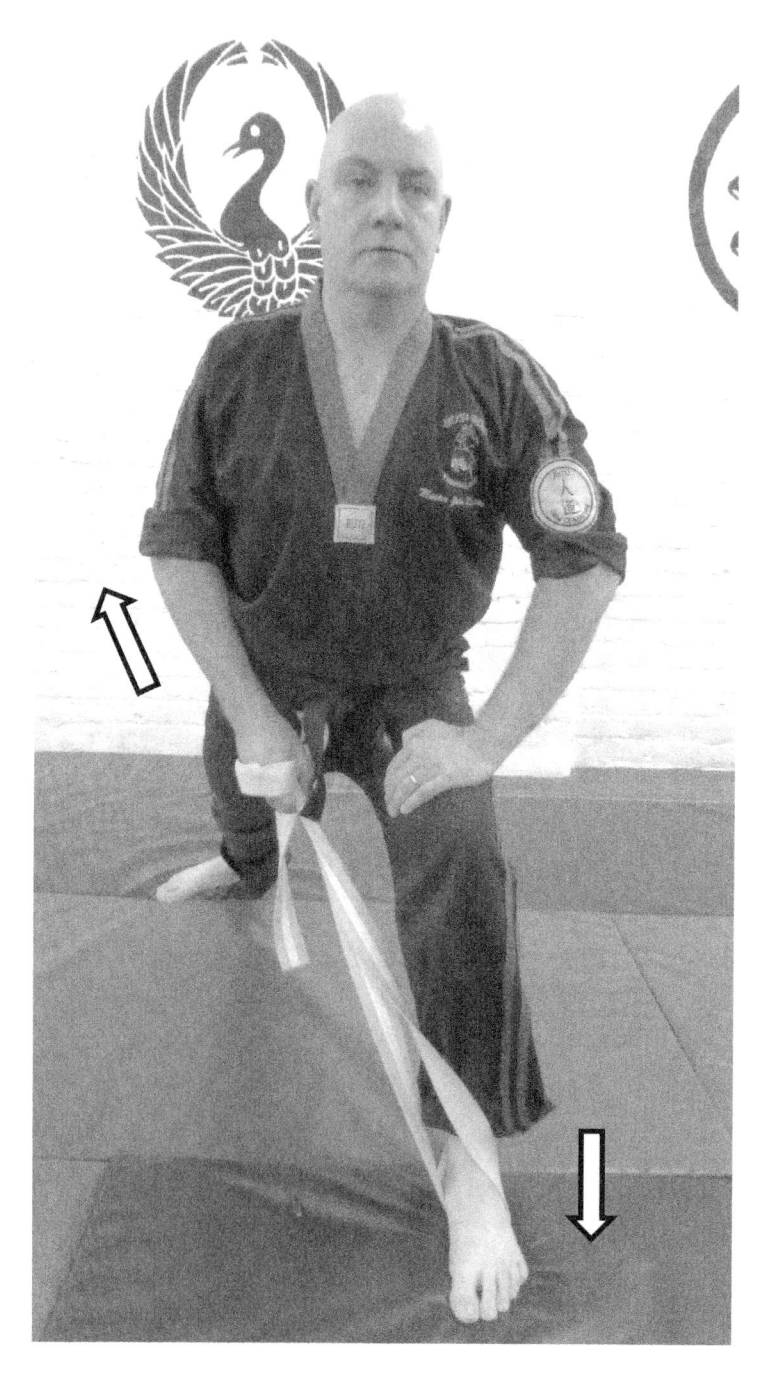

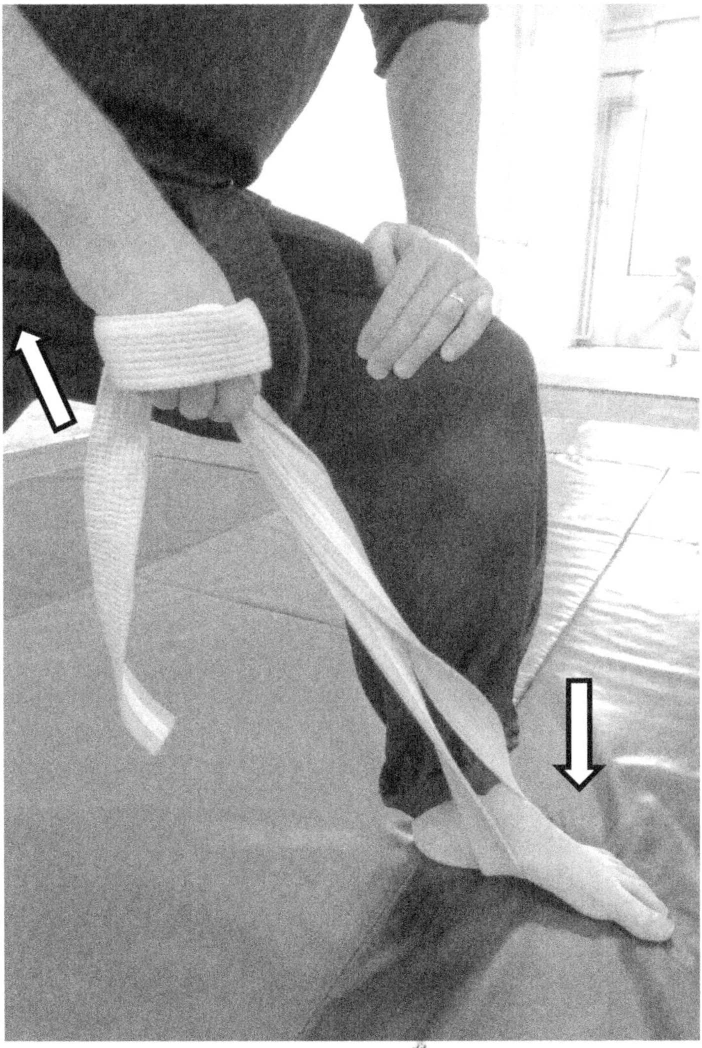

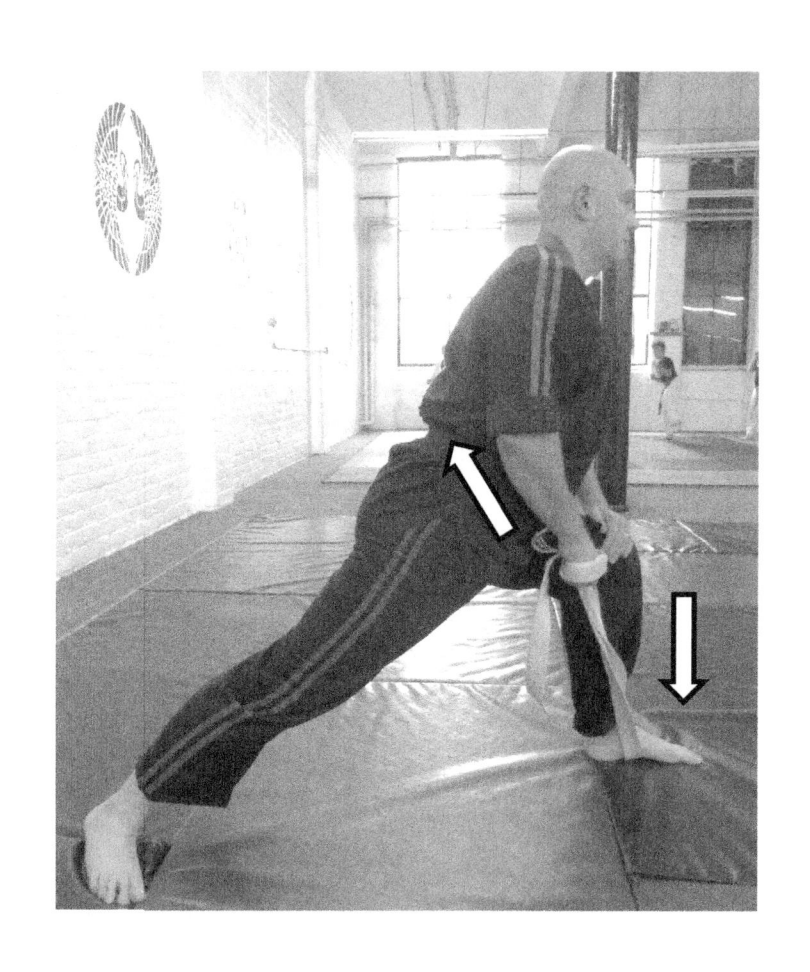

Chest – Hooking Belt Cross Press

Stand upright with your feet approximately shoulder-width apart. Hold both arms up to your front at chest level so they are parallel to the floor,

Hold an unfurled martial arts belt close together and looped around both hands. Both elbows should bend and remain locked in that position so that the arms mimic the hook punch position, but with one hook being tighter to the body than the other so they loosely interlock with each other.

The belt will be the limiting factor regarding how far each hook position is allowed to extend. In this position, apply force to mimic the hook punch using the chest muscles as the primary driver for both arms as they arc inwards with the belt providing the immovable isometric object.

When you have assumed your ideal position, hold it, and perform the isometric exercise. Be sure to change sides to exercise the chest, shoulders, and arms evenly.

The harder you engage the muscles, the more intense the exercise becomes, so always be sure to exercise at an intensity that best suits your current ability.

When you perform an isometric exercise never hold your breath. Always breathe deeply and naturally, which will be about 10 full breaths in and out at a rate of about 1 second per full breath. Perform each exercise for no less than 7 seconds, and no longer than 10.

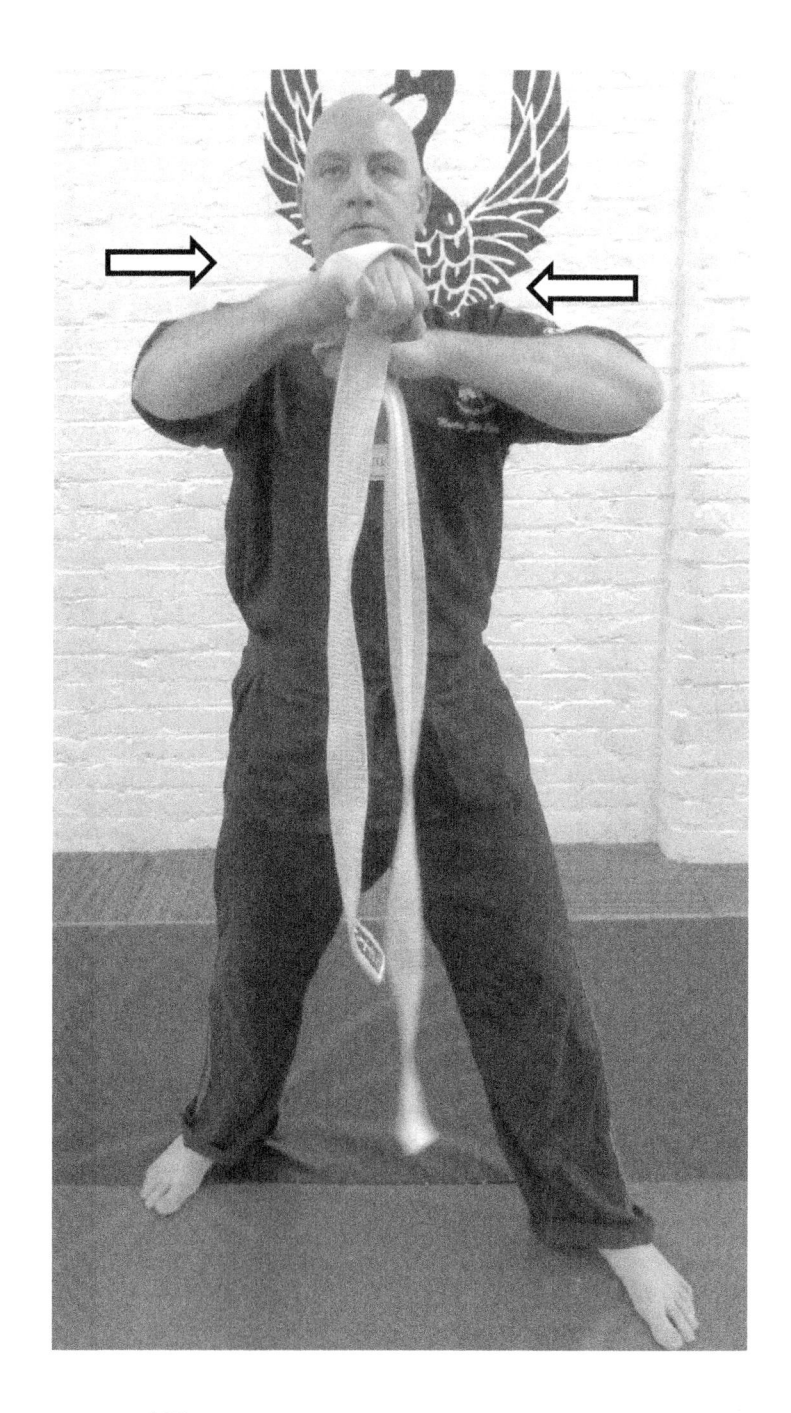

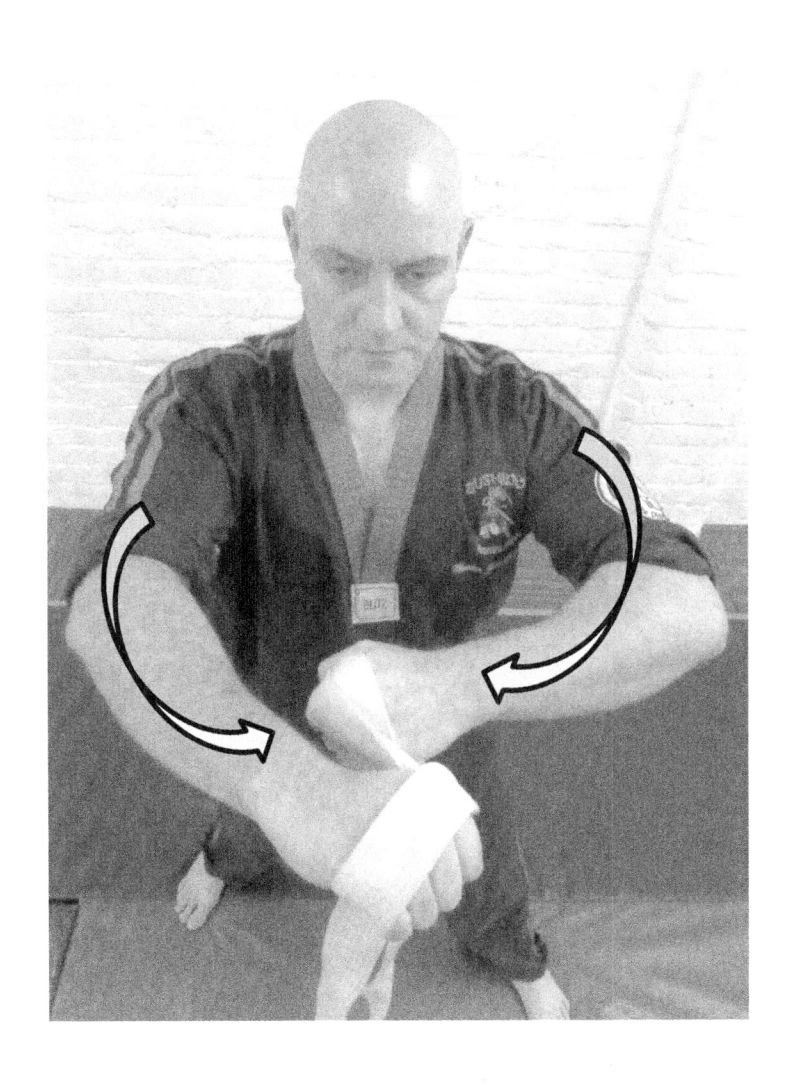

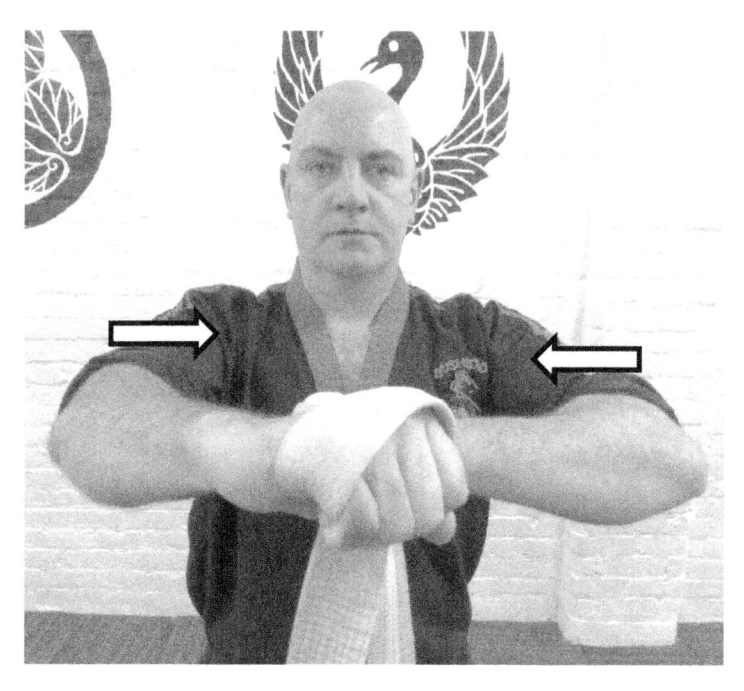

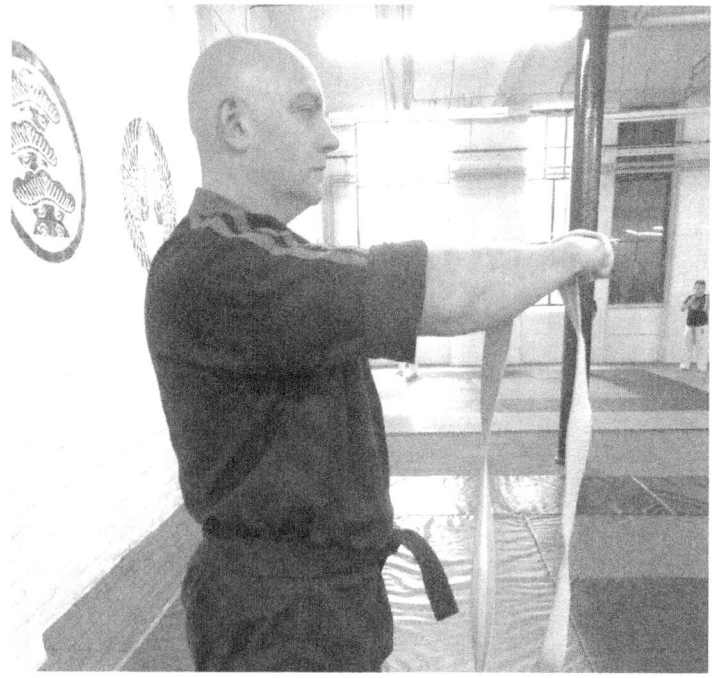

Chest – Partner Hands Interlocked Cross Press

To perform this exercise both partners stand upright facing each other at a close distance. They both hold their arms and hands at chest height so their hands meet and fingers can interlock if necessary.

This means that the right hand of one partner interlocks palms with the right hand of the other partner, and the left hands assume the same type of interlock.

In this position, the forearms should be horizontal to the floor and the elbows raised to the side. Both partners press inwards with each resisting the other simultaneously pressing an interlocked palm against palm. This will engage the chest muscles.

When you have assumed your ideal position, hold it, and perform the isometric exercise.

Be sure to change sides to exercise the chest, shoulders, and arms evenly.

Be sure to swap hands over after performing one isometric exercise to exercise both sides of the chest evenly.

The harder you engage the muscles, the more intense the exercise becomes, so always be sure to exercise at an intensity that best suits your current ability. When you perform an isometric exercise never hold your breath.

Always breathe deeply and naturally, which will be about 10 full breaths in and out at a rate of about 1 second per full breath. Perform each exercise for no less than 7 seconds, and no longer than 10.

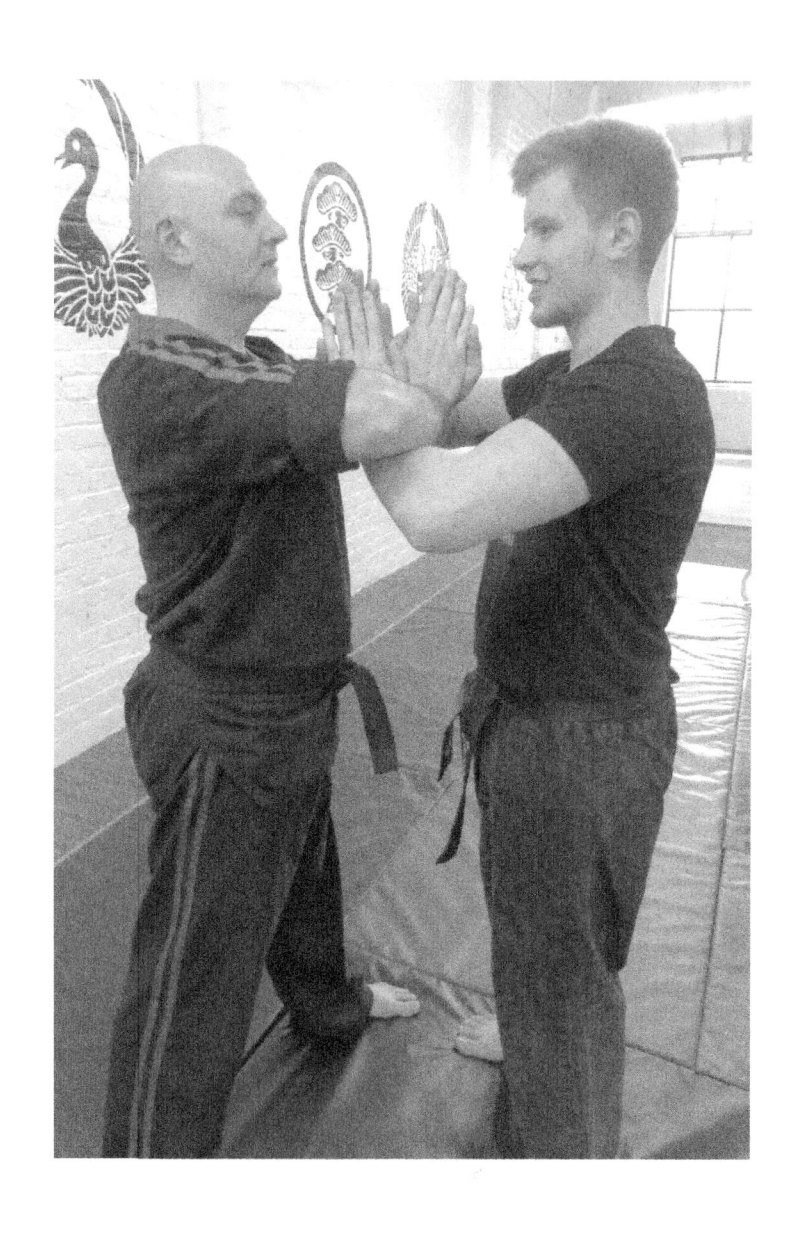

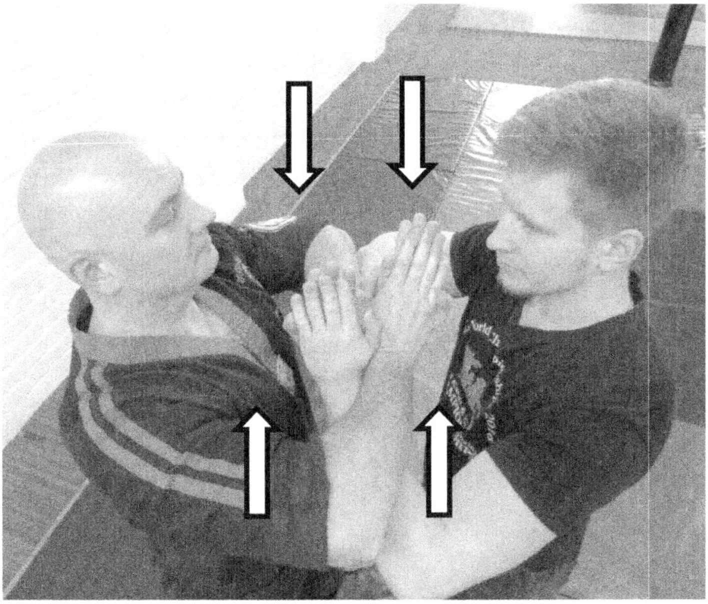

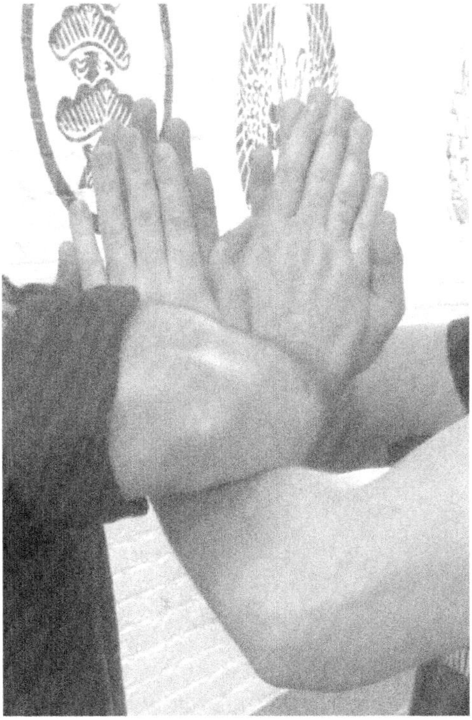

Chest – Hand-Palm Press Cross Press Variation

This is a variation of the partner-based exercise that can be performed alone. Instead of interlocking hands with a partner, simply press the palms of your hands together evenly at the midpoint of the chest. Be sure to keep your elbows high and your upper arms parallel to the floor throughout the exercise. Perform the standard isometric exercise in the same way as before.

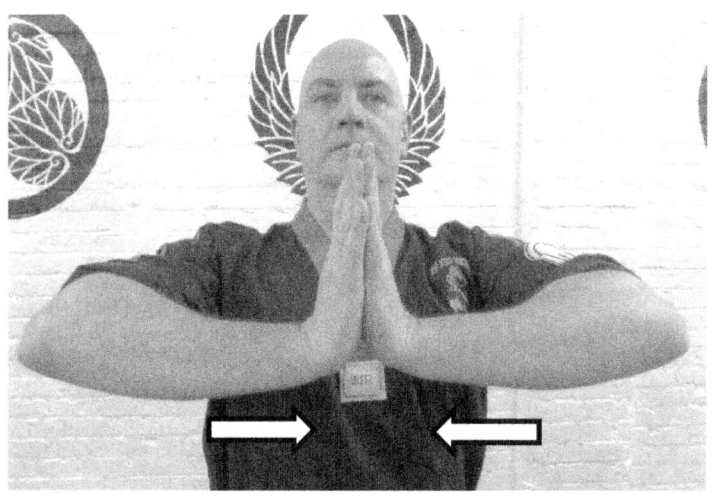

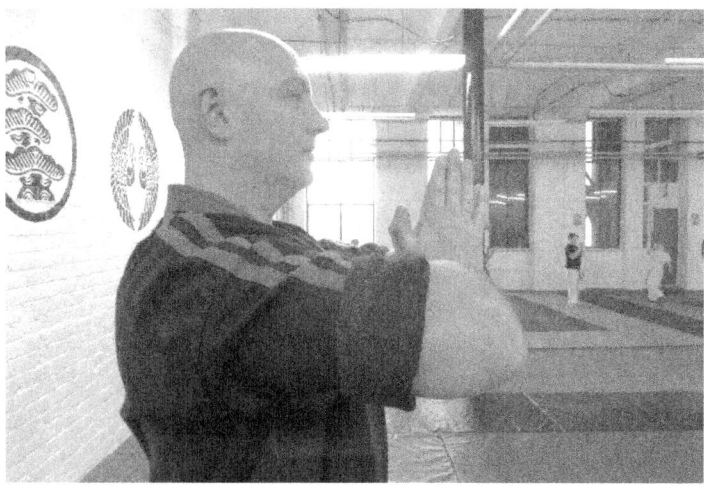

Chest – Push-up Hold

Perform a standard push-up from the mat or floor. Place the hands on the mat wider than shoulder-width apart and with your upper arms out to the side to create a letter 'T' shape with your body if viewed from above.

Make sure the hand position is wide enough to create a 90-degree angle between the upper arm and forearm at the mid-bend position.

Push up from the floor slowly to assume the midpoint position and perform then perform the standard isometric exercise.

The harder you engage the muscles, the more intense the exercise becomes, so always be sure to exercise at an intensity that best suits your current ability. When you perform an isometric exercise never hold your breath.

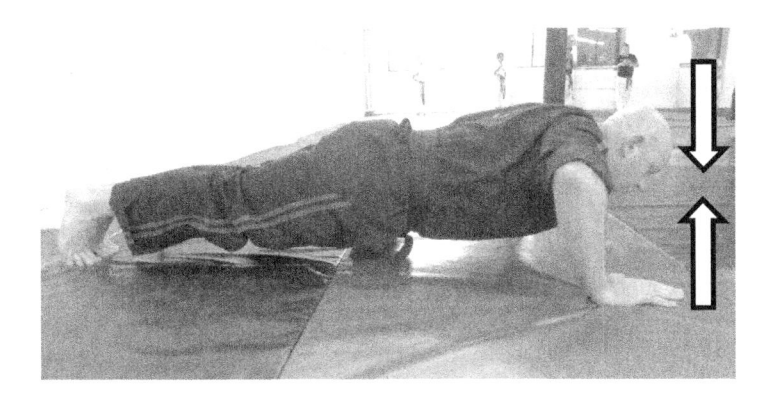

Always breathe deeply and naturally, which will be about 10 full breaths in and out at a rate of about 1 second per full breath. Perform each exercise for no less than 7 seconds, and no longer than 10.

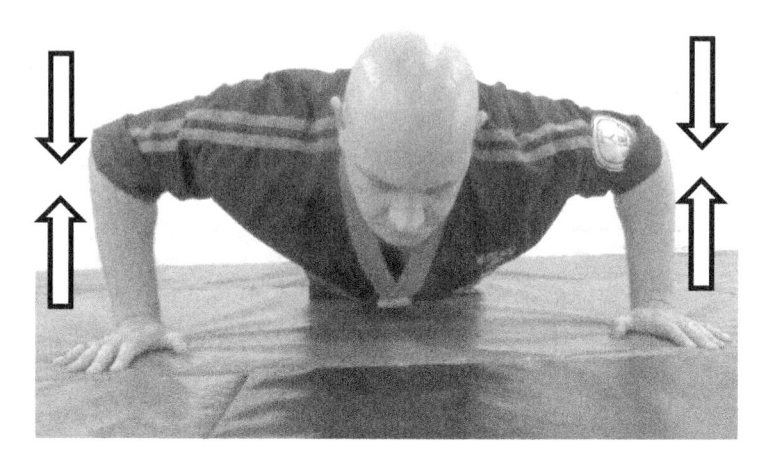

Chest – Push-up Hold Belt Resisted Variation

This variation is performed in the same way as the standard push-up hold, except that an unfurled martial arts belt is wrapped around the shoulders and upper back, and then looped around the hands to provide immovable resistance. This is a more advanced exercise than the version without the belt. Perform the standard isometric exercise in the same way as before.

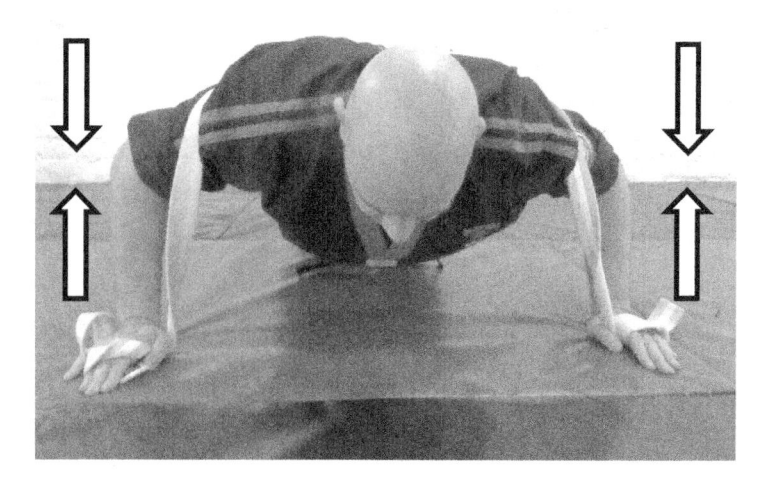

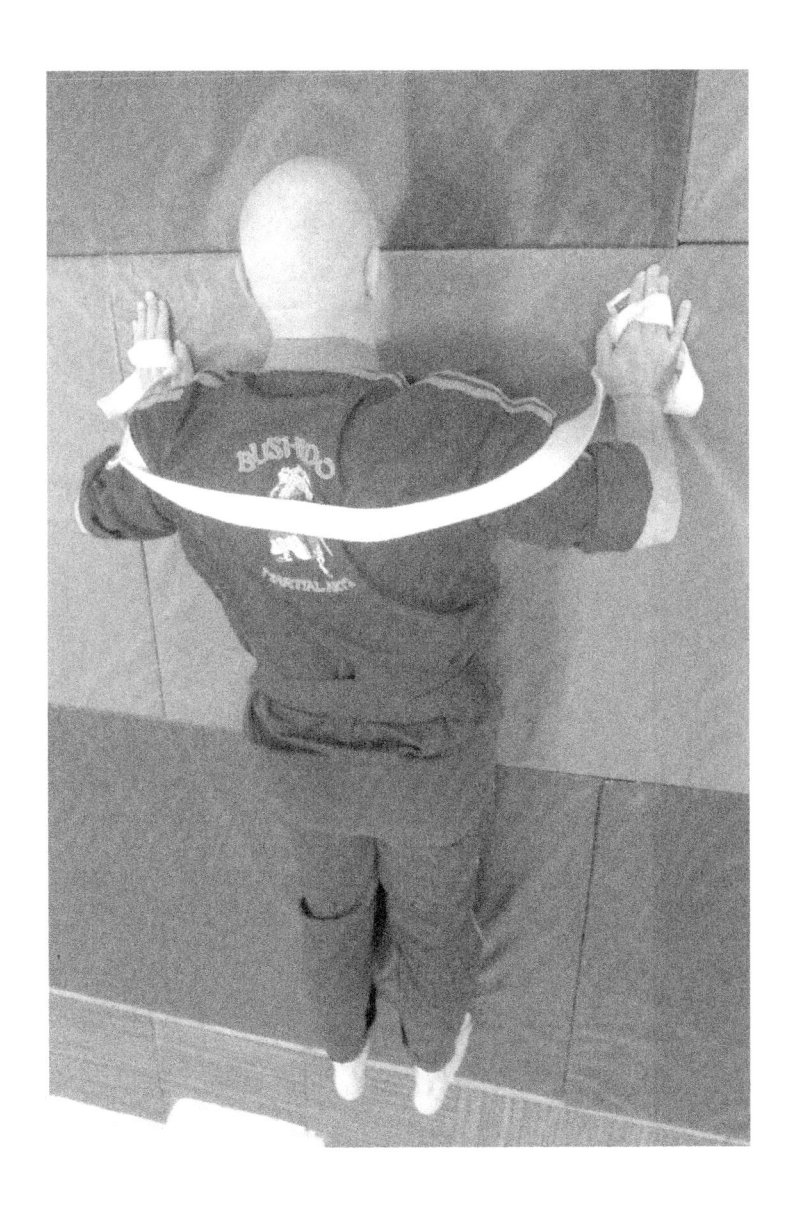
BUSHIDO

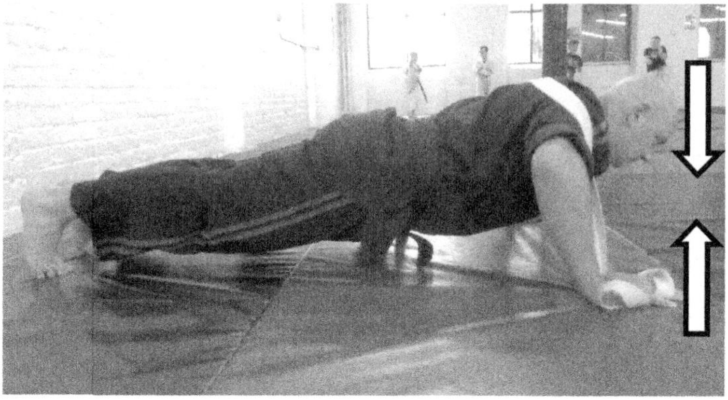

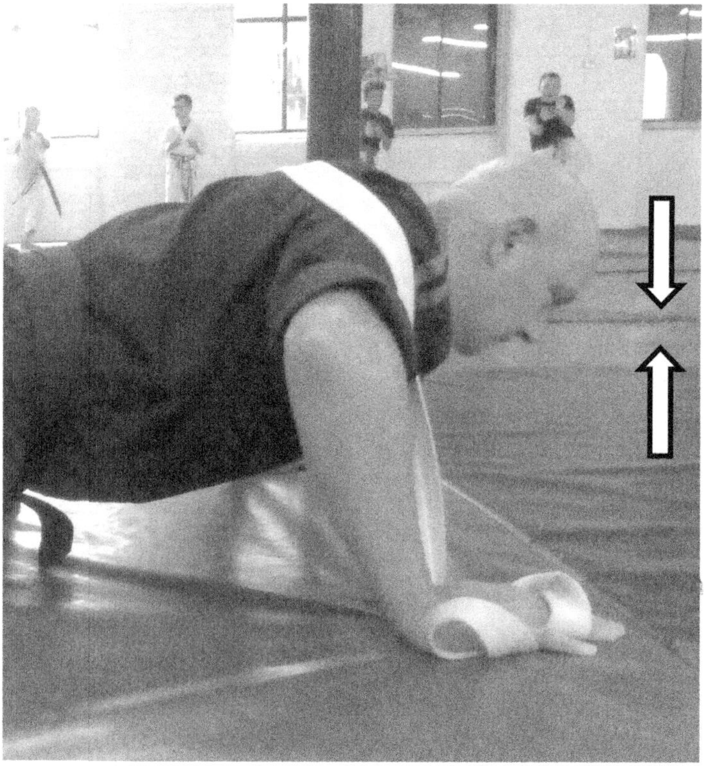

Legs – Calf's – Double Heel Raise Wall Push

Stand upright, lean forward, and press your hands against a wall or any other completely solid immovable object. In this position, attempt to move the immovable object by using the force generated by the calf muscles when performing a double heel raise.

Be sure to position yourself so that you are at approximately the mid-heel raised position when you begin the isometric exercise and apply maximum force.

The harder you engage the muscles, the more intense the exercise becomes, so always be sure to exercise at an intensity that best suits your current ability. When you perform an isometric exercise never hold your breath.

Always breathe deeply and naturally, which will be about 10 full breaths in and out at a rate of about 1 second per full breath. Perform each exercise for no less than 7 seconds, and no longer than 10.

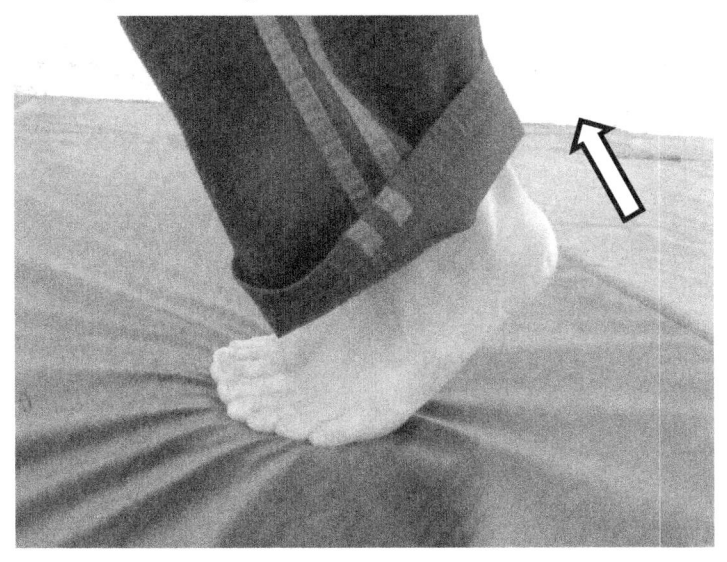

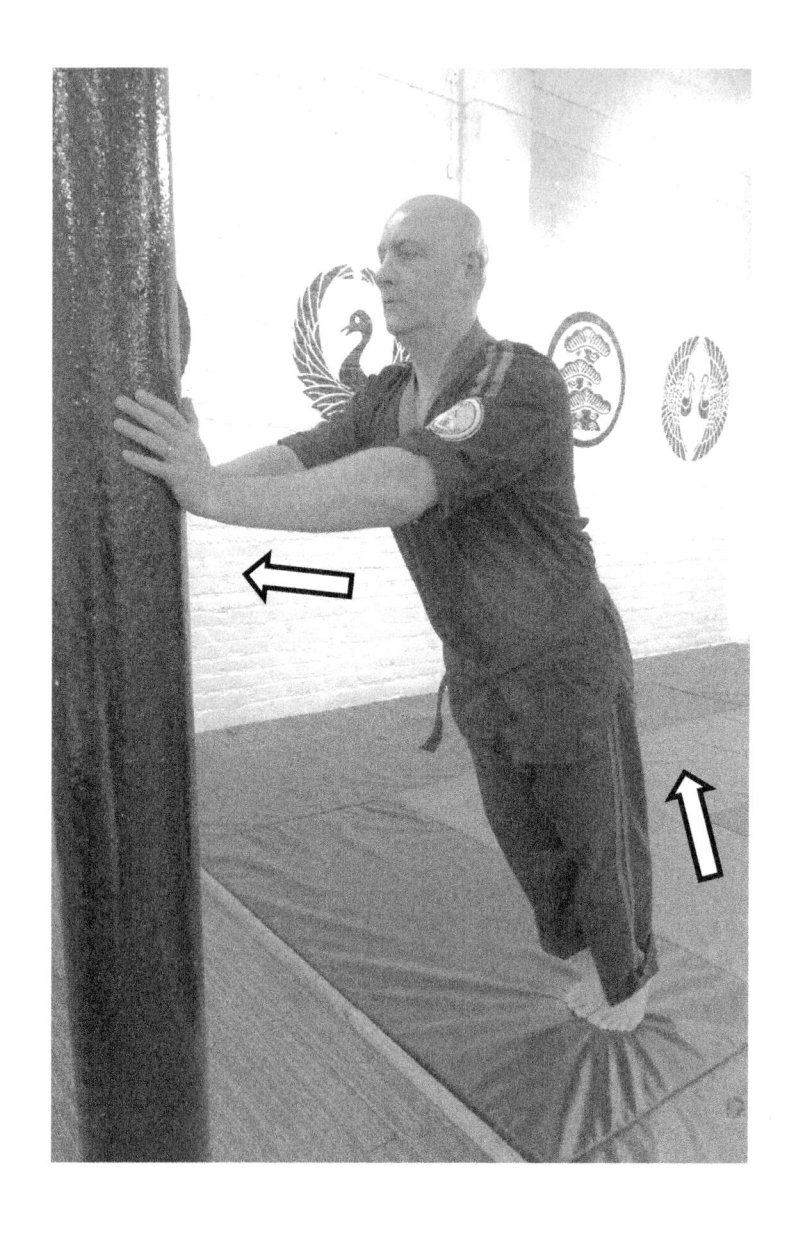

Legs – Calf's
Single Heel Raise Wall Push Variation

The single heel raise is essentially performed in exactly the same way as the double heel raise exercise, with the only difference being that one leg is exercised instead of two.

When performing the single heel raise, tuck the other resting leg/foot neatly away by wrapping it close to the leg being exercised.

Be sure to change over and exercise both legs evenly. Perform the standard isometric exercise in the same way as before.

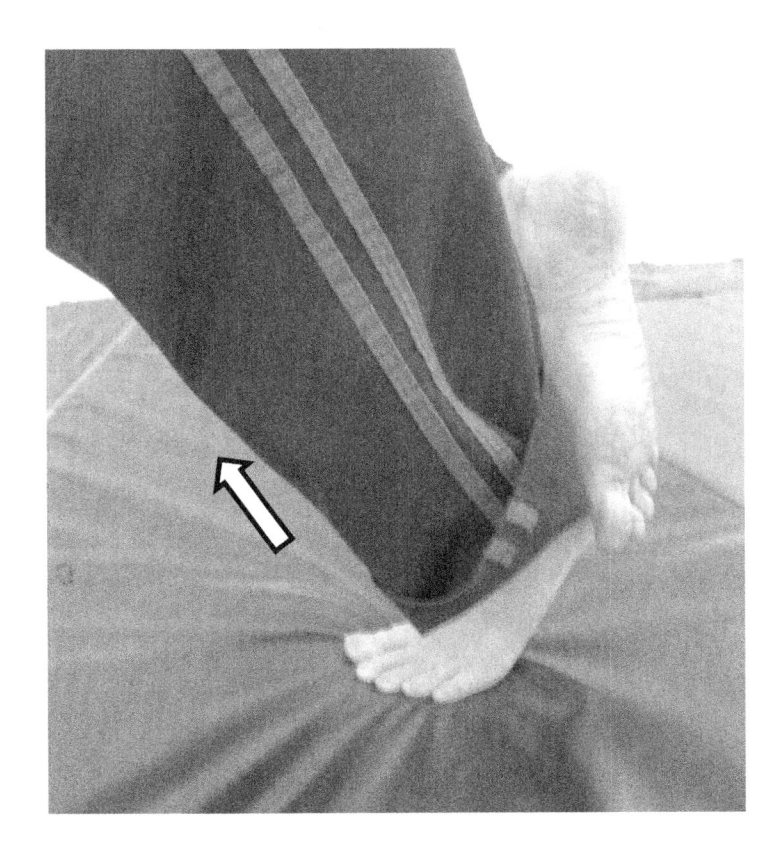

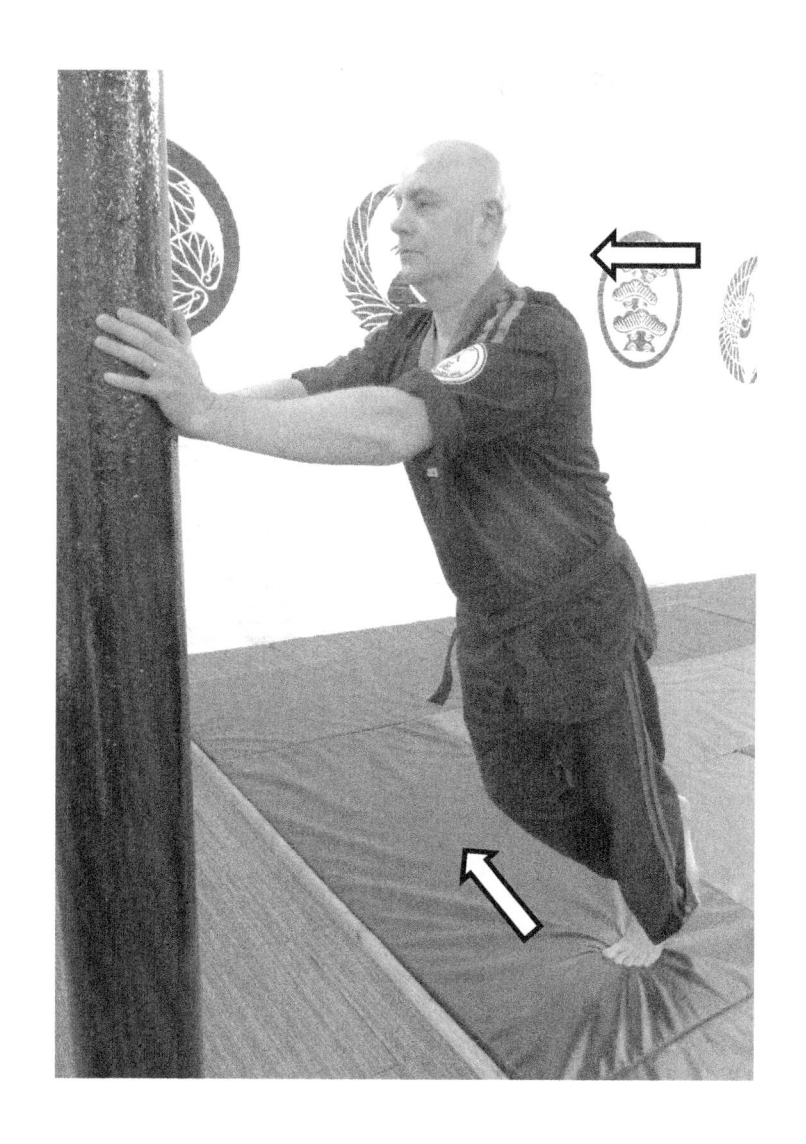

Legs – Single Leg Belt Extension

This exercise mimics the action of extending the lower leg during a variety of front kicks. Sit on a chair, bench, or any other solid object. Raise one leg with a bent knee. Wrap an unfurled martial arts belt flat around the lower shin, close to the foot. Grip the other two ends of the belt by looping them around both hands. In this position, generate force by attempting to extend the lower leg forwards, to straighten it in the same way as if performing a front kick. Be sure to allow enough belt room to prevent the leg from moving further than the approximate midpoint position. Perform the standard isometric exercise. Be sure to change over and exercise both legs evenly. The harder you engage the muscles, the more intense the exercise becomes, so always be sure to exercise at an intensity that best suits your current ability. When you perform an isometric exercise never hold your breath. Always breathe deeply and naturally at about 10 full breaths in and out at a rate of about 1 second per full breath. Perform each exercise for no less than 7 seconds, and no longer than 10.

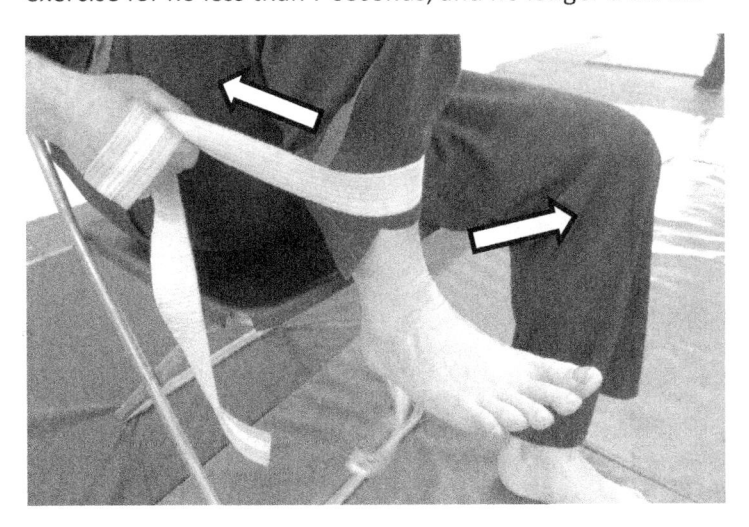

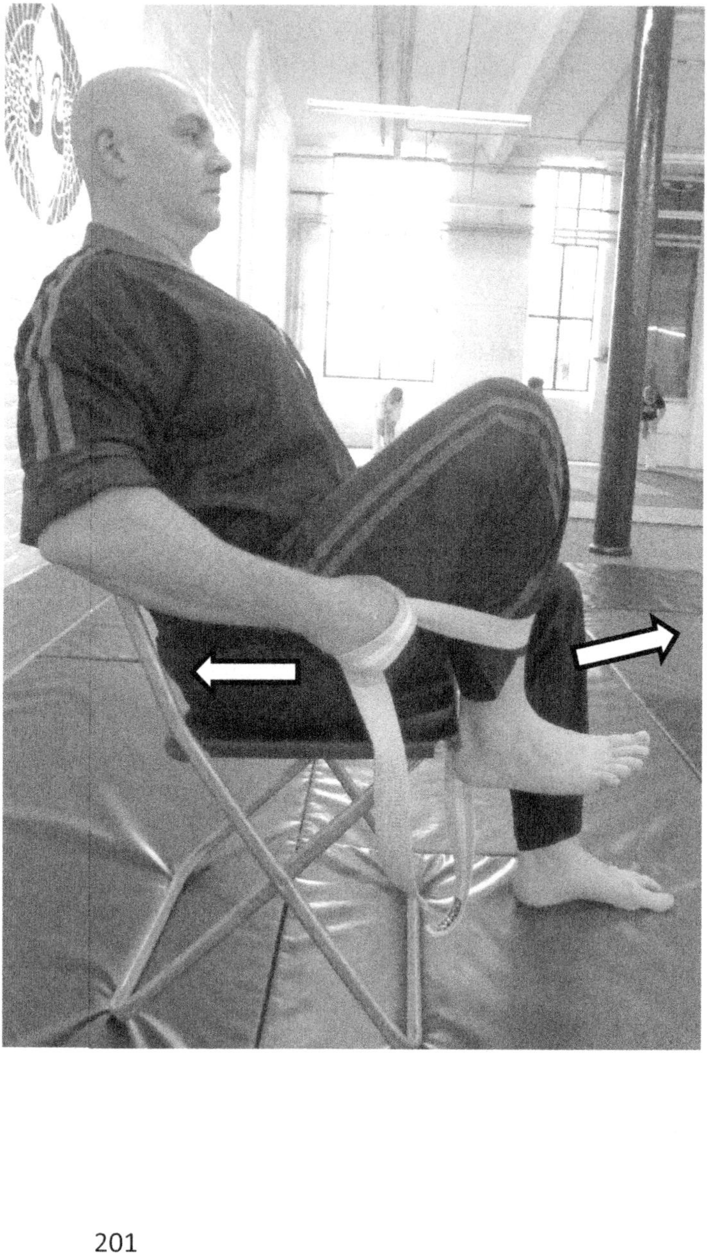

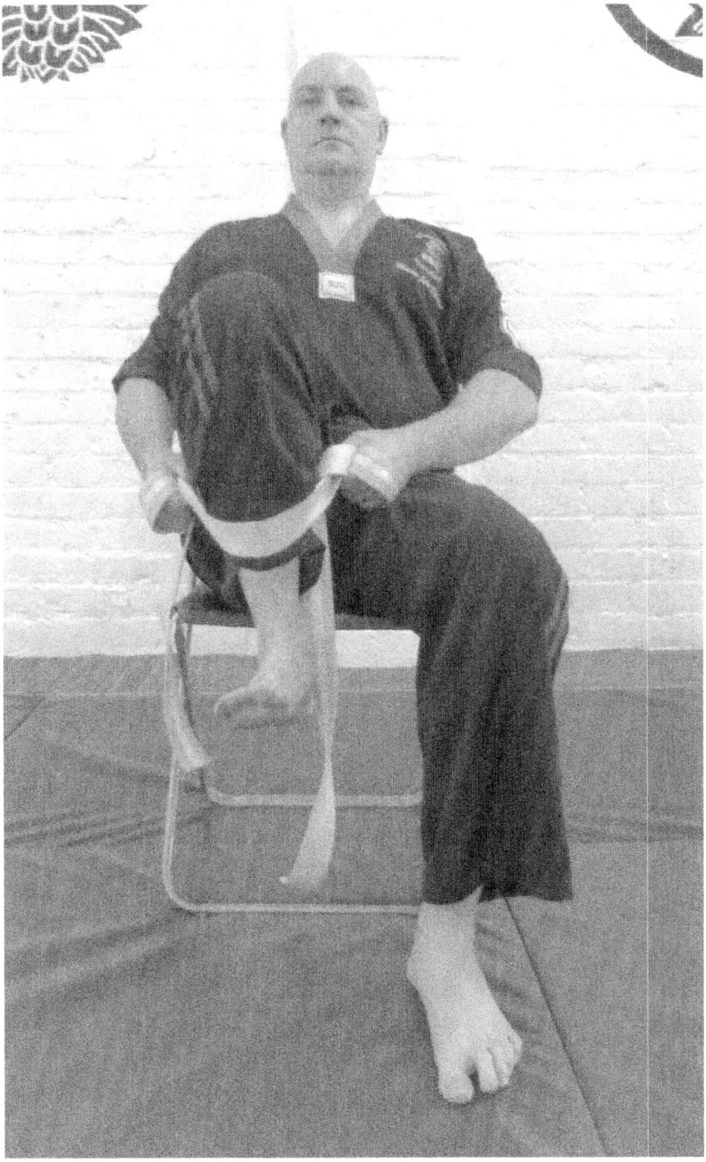

Legs – Single Leg Hand Wrap Extension Variation

This exercise is performed in the same way as the previous exercise with the exception being that instead of a martial arts belt being used to provide immovable resistance, the hands are used instead.

This is done by wrapping both hands around the lower shin to prevent the lower leg from moving past any desired position you choose.

Once your ideal exercise position has been attained, then perform the standard isometric exercise.

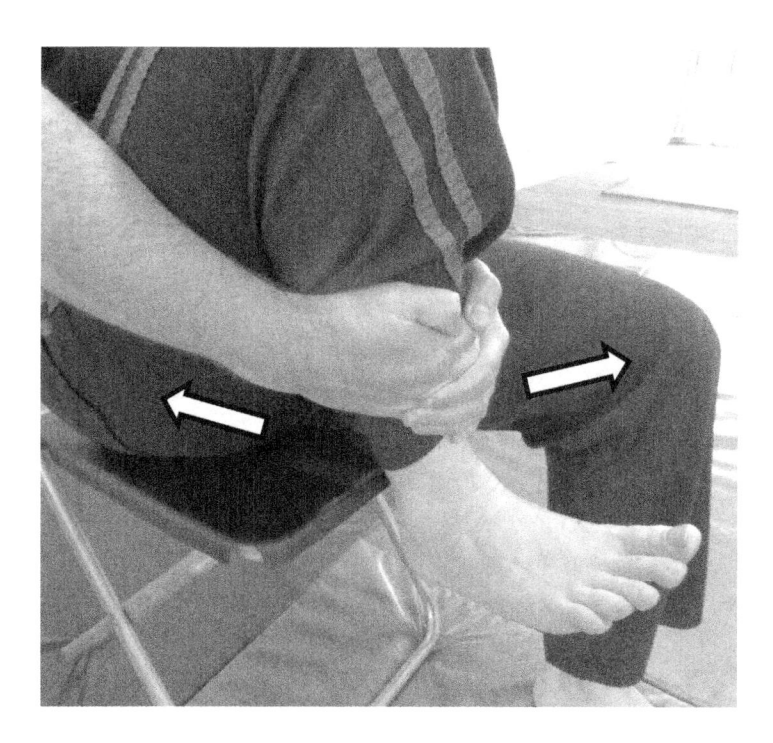

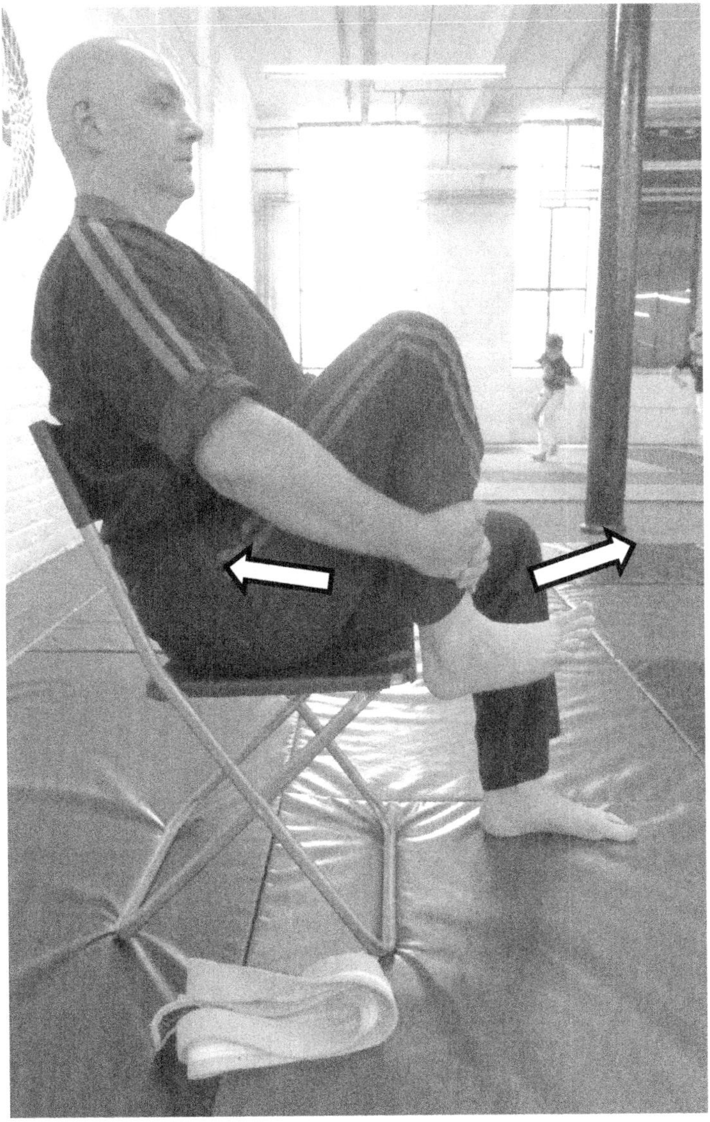

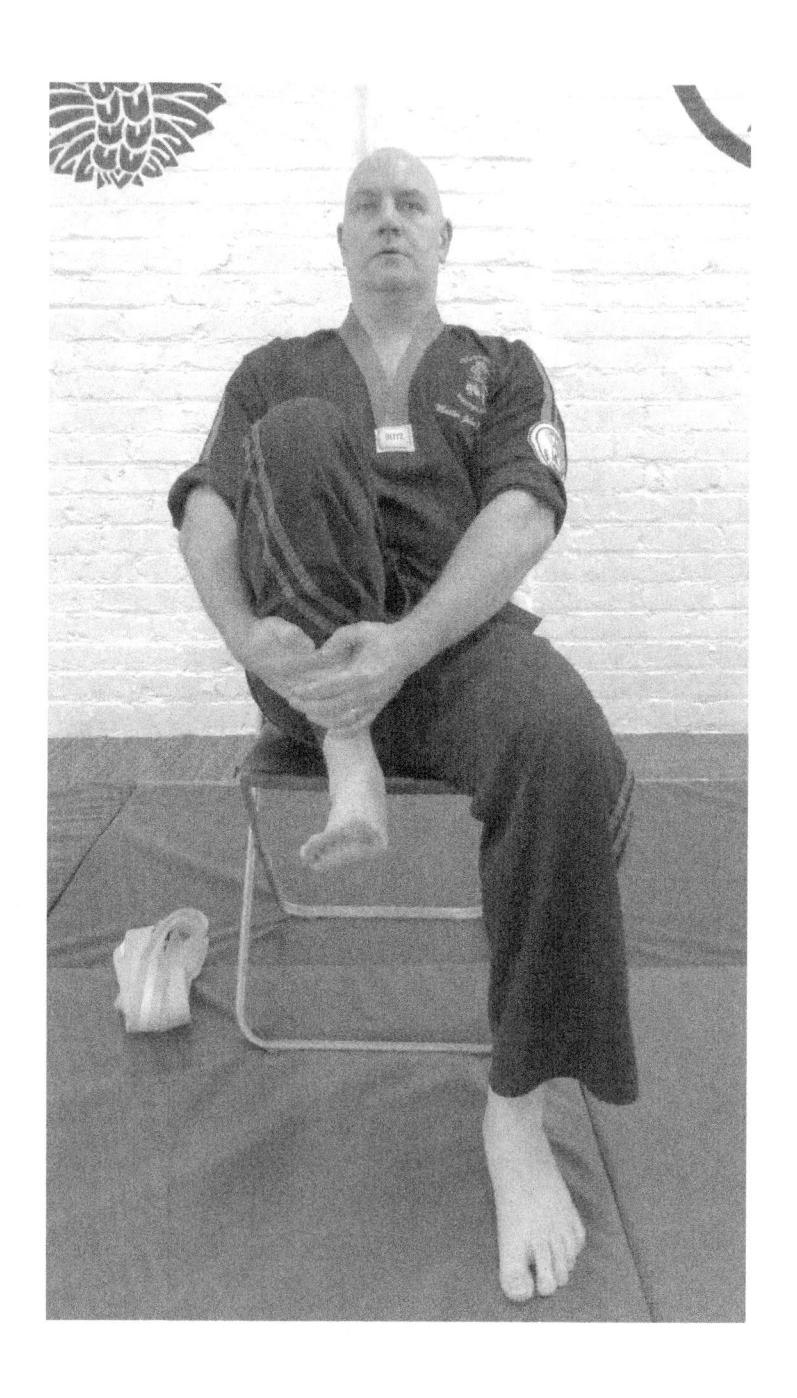

Legs – Partner Leg Press

One partner lies flat on the floor with both legs raised in the 'baby' position. The other partner stands in front of their legs. They then connect with the partner on the floor extending their legs to meet the upright partner as they lean forward to rest on the feet of the floor-based partner. In this position, the standing/leaning partner places their weight on the feet/legs of the floor-based partner. However, both parties should always be ready in case one or both of the partners fail at any time during the exercise causing one to fall etc. Therefore, always perform this exercise with caution, on a well-padded mat and with great caution. The exercising partner is the partner on the floor, and once the weight of the upper partner has been taken by the floor-based partner's legs, then the floor-based partner bends their legs in a leg press action to a point where an isometric exercise can be performed.

NOTE: the floor-based partner can always help to brace their legs if needed by using their hands on their knees/upper thighs for support. Once your ideal exercise position has been attained, then perform the standard isometric exercise.

The harder you engage the muscles, the more intense the exercise becomes, so always be sure to exercise at an intensity that best suits your current ability. When you perform an isometric exercise never hold your breath.

Always breathe deeply and naturally, which will be about 10 full breaths in and out at a rate of about 1 second per full breath. Perform each exercise for no less than 7 seconds, and no longer than 10.

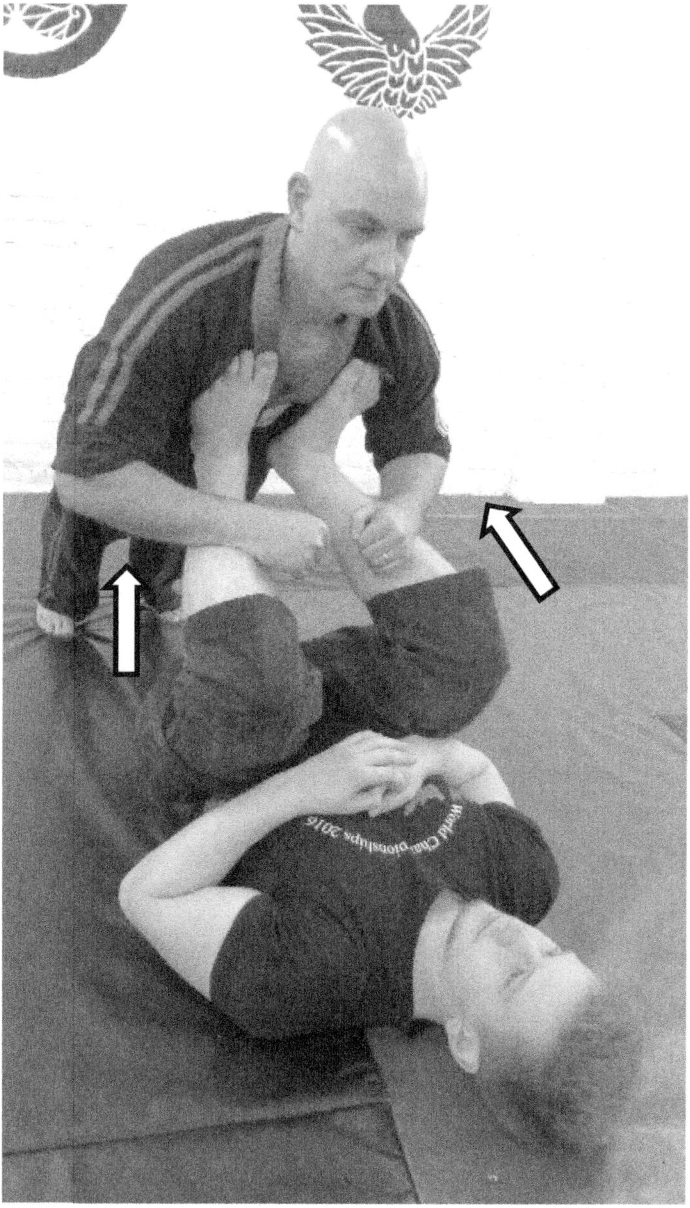

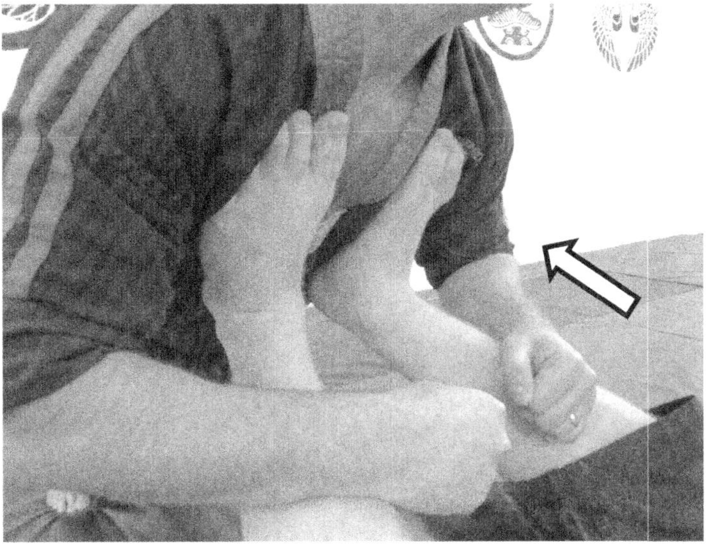

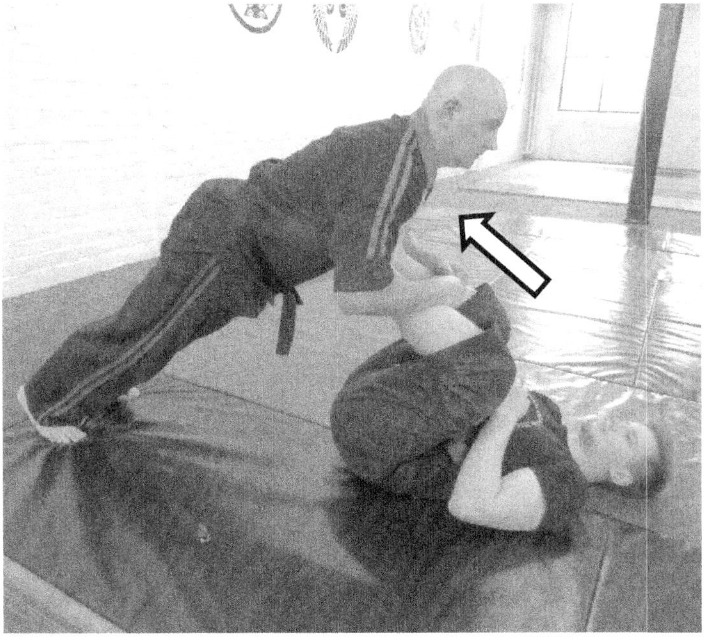

Legs – Split Squat Hold

Stand upright on a mat, then step squarely forward with one leg into a forward stance position. It does not matter which leg is used first as both will be exercised during the workout session. The forward leg should then perform a controlled deep knee bend into a split squat position. At the lowest part of the split squat, the rear leg/knee should never quite touch the floor. In this position, use the thigh muscles to maintain the exercise point to perform the isometric exercise. Remember to exercise both legs the same way. The harder you engage the muscles, the more intense the exercise becomes, so always be sure to exercise at an intensity that best suits your current ability. When you perform an isometric exercise never hold your breath. Always breathe deeply and naturally, which will be about 10 full breaths in and out at a rate of about 1 second per full breath. Perform each exercise for no less than 7 seconds, and no longer than 10.

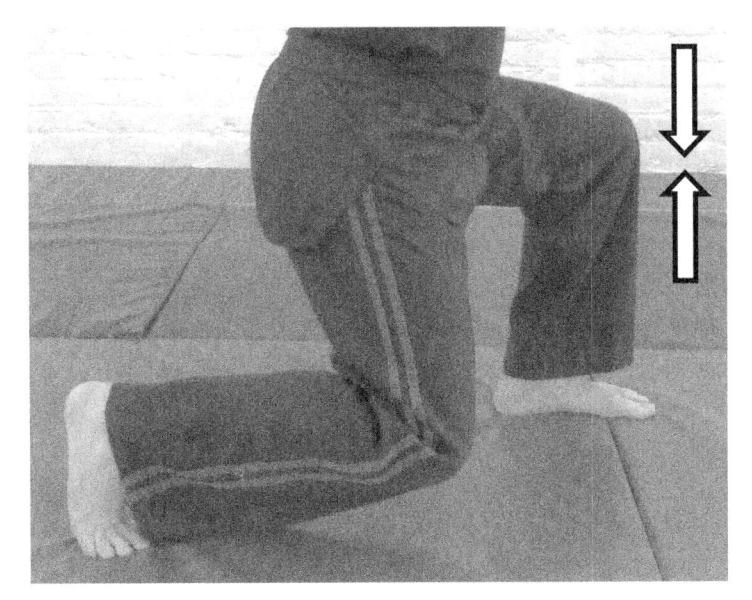

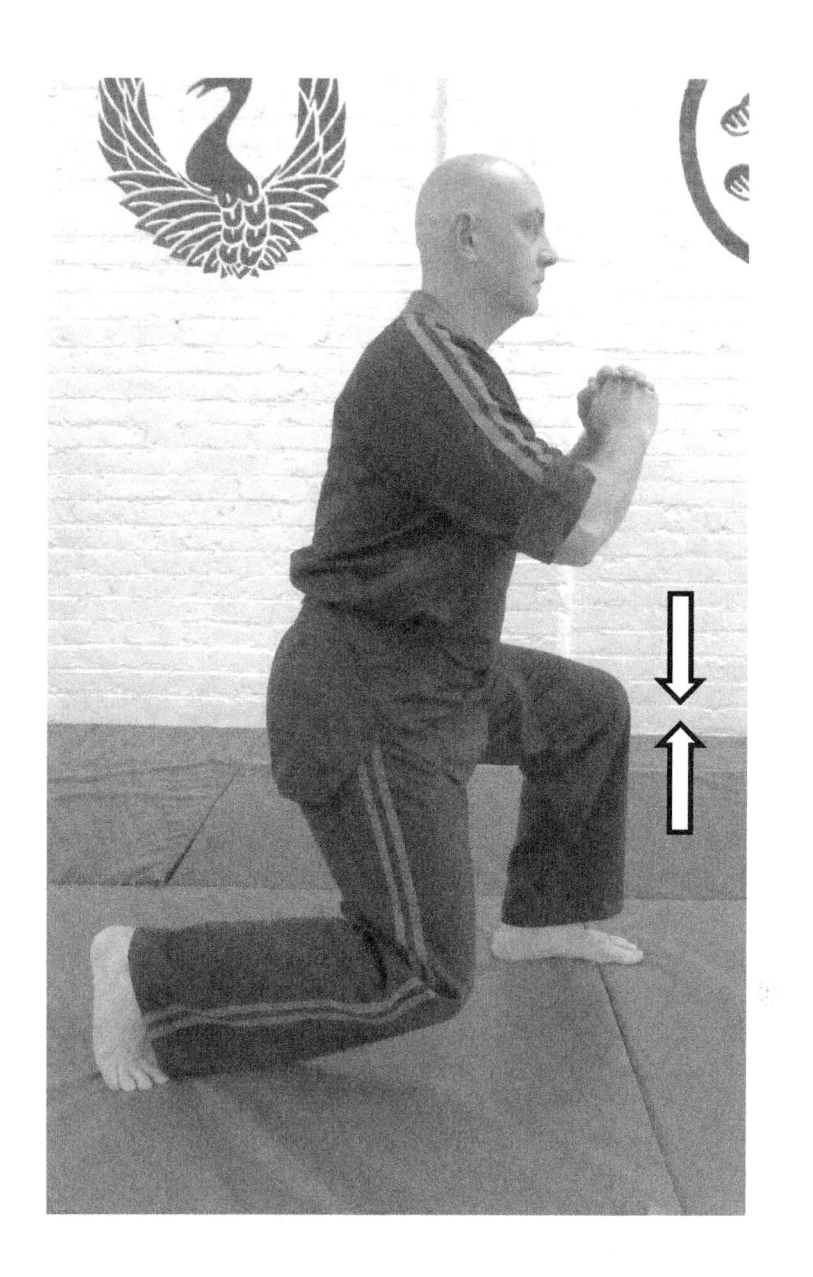

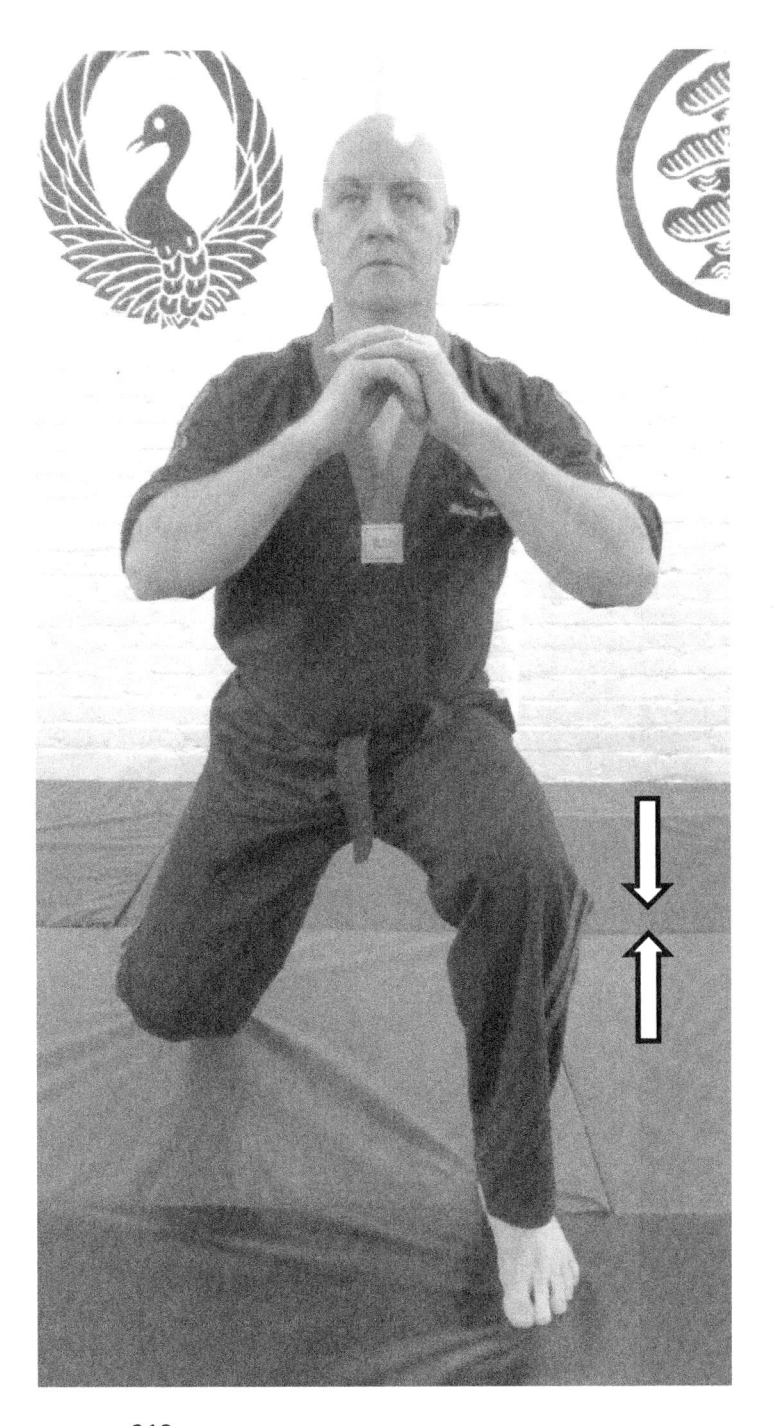

Legs – Split Squat Belt Hold Variation

This variation is performed in the same way as the previous split squat exercise except that it uses a martial arts belt to provide immovable resistance. This is achieved by the front lunging leg standing on an evenly unfurled belt. As the knee bends into the split squat position, the belt is held and wrapped around the hands so that when force is generated to stand up from the lower split squat position the belt provides an immovable resistance. The standard isometric is performed in the same way.

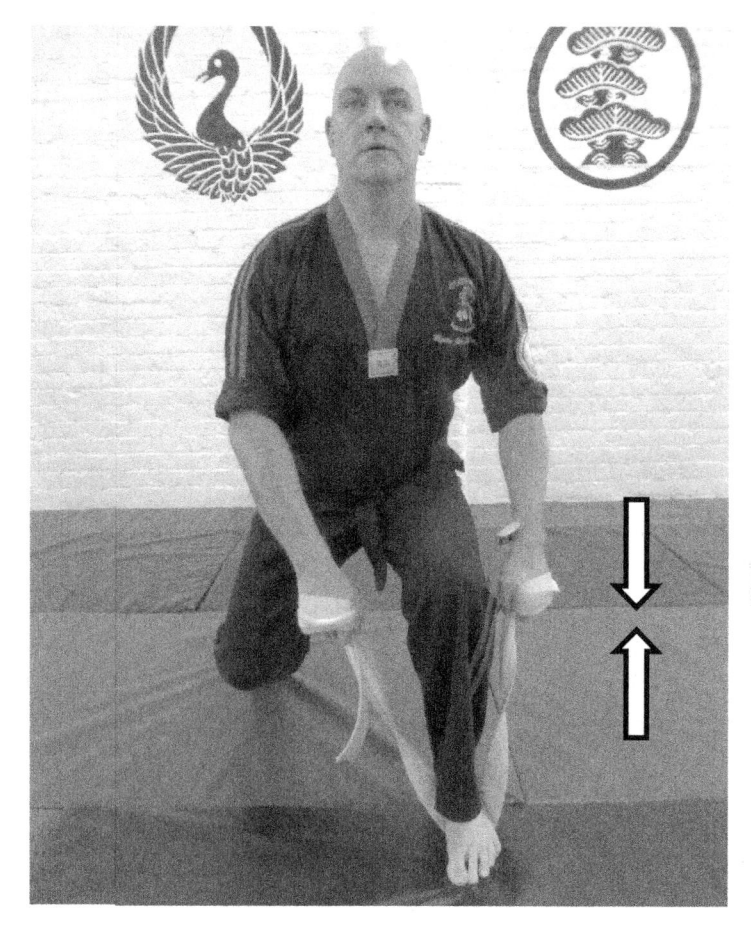

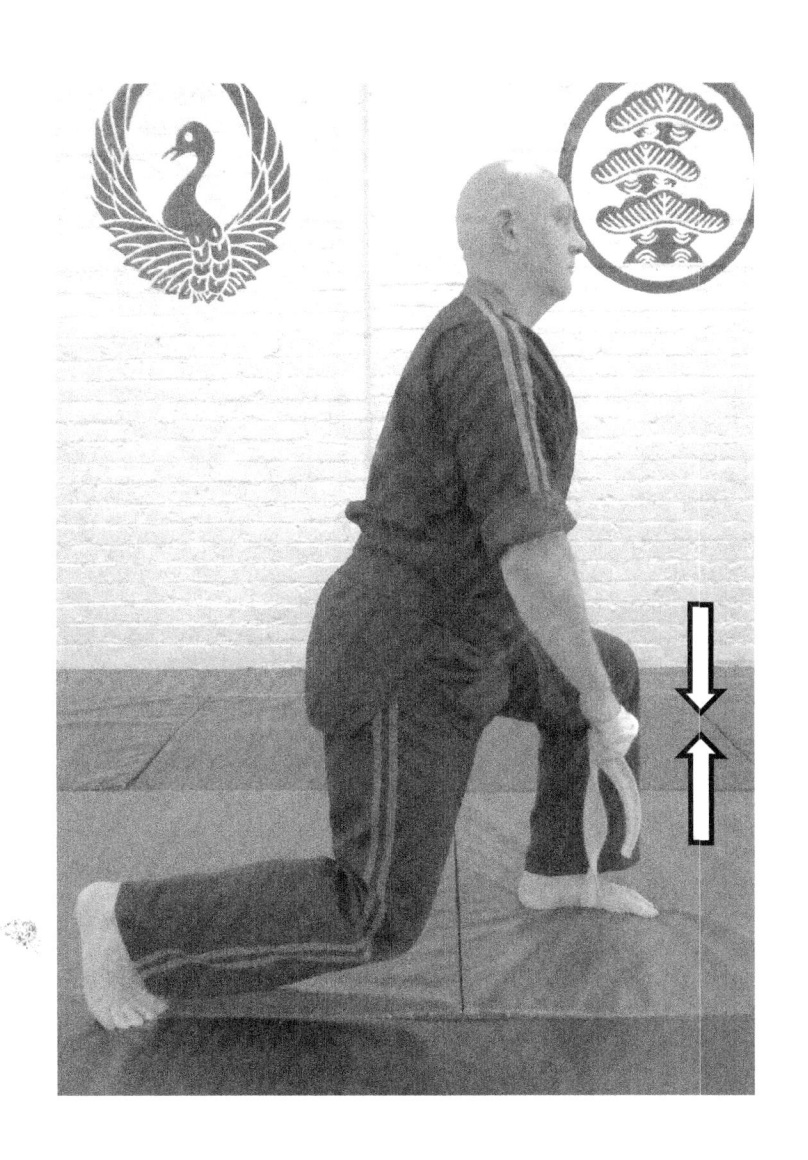

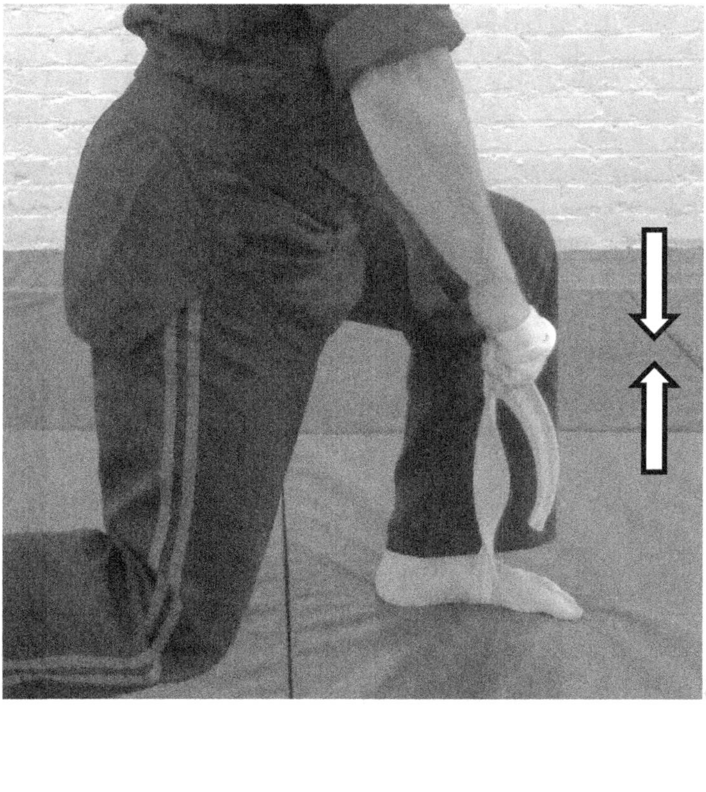

Legs – Leaning Belt Squat Hold

      Secure an unfurled martial arts belt around a solid pillar or any other similar immovable object that is safe to use. Hold the belt at approximately equal length and loop both ends around each hand. Bend the knees into a squat position so that your upper thighs are parallel to the floor. Lean back to support yourself on the belt as you do so. Always bend from the hips and keep the back straight. Once you have assumed your ideal leaning squat hold position, then perform the isometric exercise.

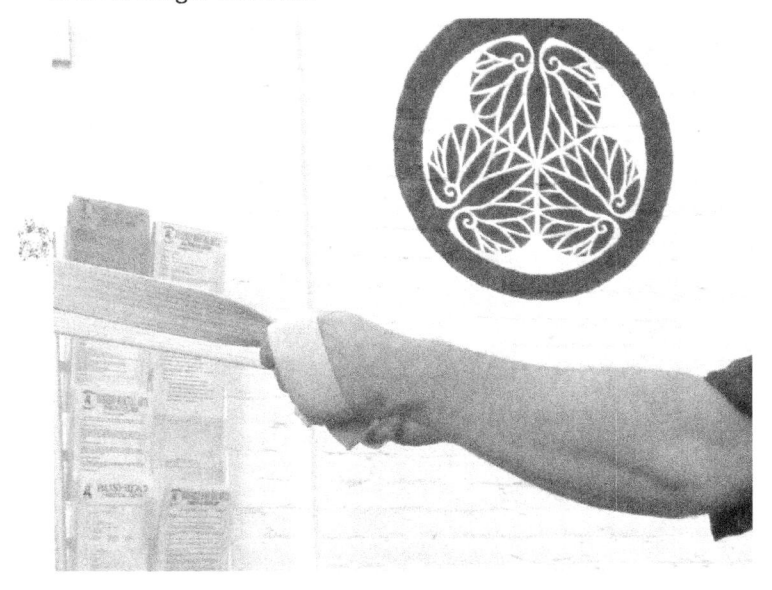

      The harder you engage the muscles, the more intense the exercise becomes, so always be sure to exercise at an intensity that best suits your current ability. When you perform an isometric exercise never hold your breath. Always breathe deeply and naturally, which will be about 10 full breaths in and out at a rate of about 1 second per full breath. Perform each exercise for no less than 7 seconds, and no longer than 10.

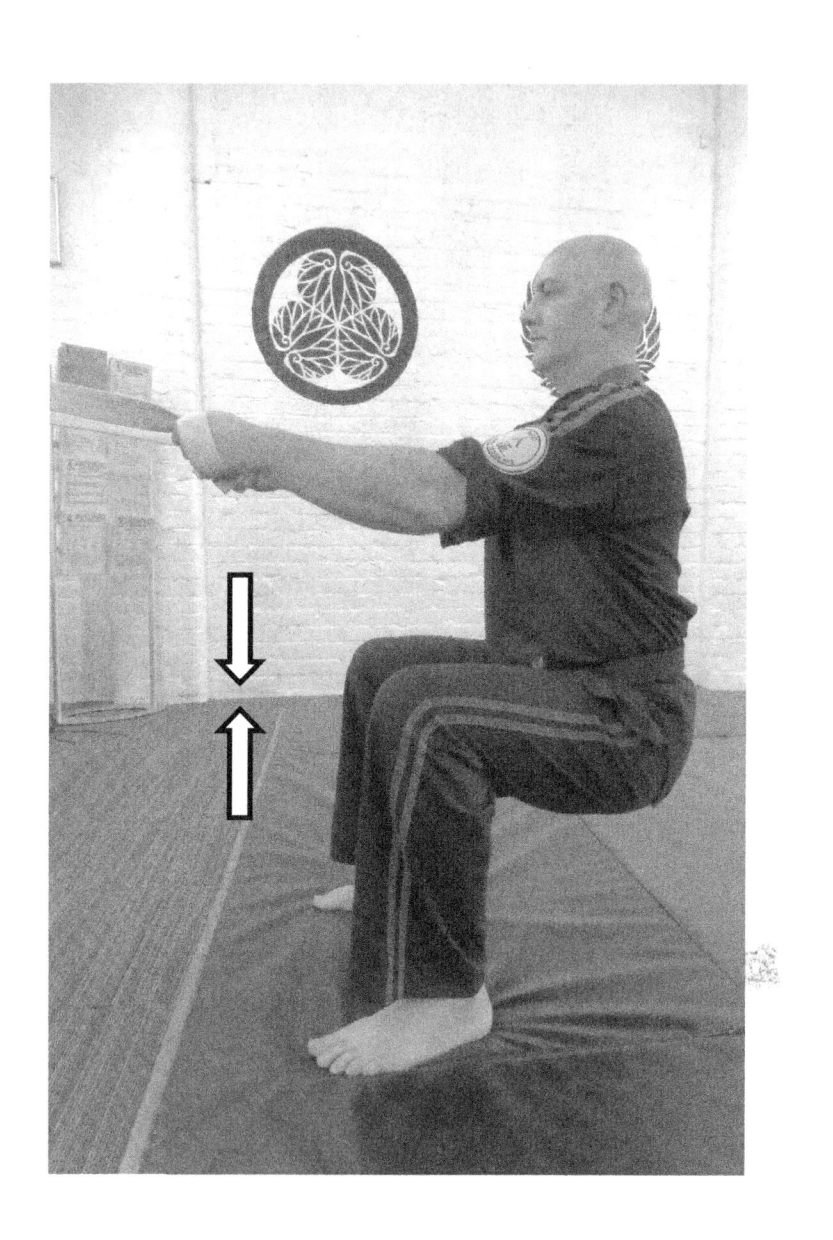

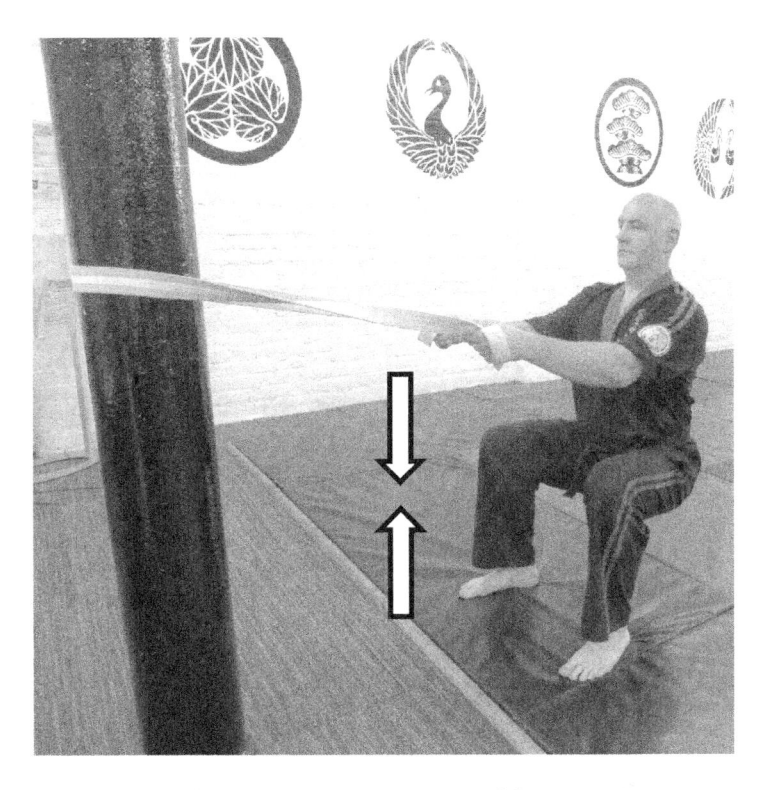

Leaning Belt Single-Leg Squat Hold Variation

Secure an unfurled martial arts belt around a solid pillar or any other similar immovable object that is safe to use. Hold the belt at approximately equal length and loop both ends around each hand. Bend one knee into a single-leg squat position so that your upper thigh is parallel to the floor. Lean back to support yourself on the belt as you do so. Tuck your other leg out of the way or hold it forward and away from the floor. Always bend from the hips and keep the back straight. Once you have assumed your ideal leaning squat hold position, then perform the isometric exercise as before. Be sure to exercise both sides of the body by changing sides etc

219

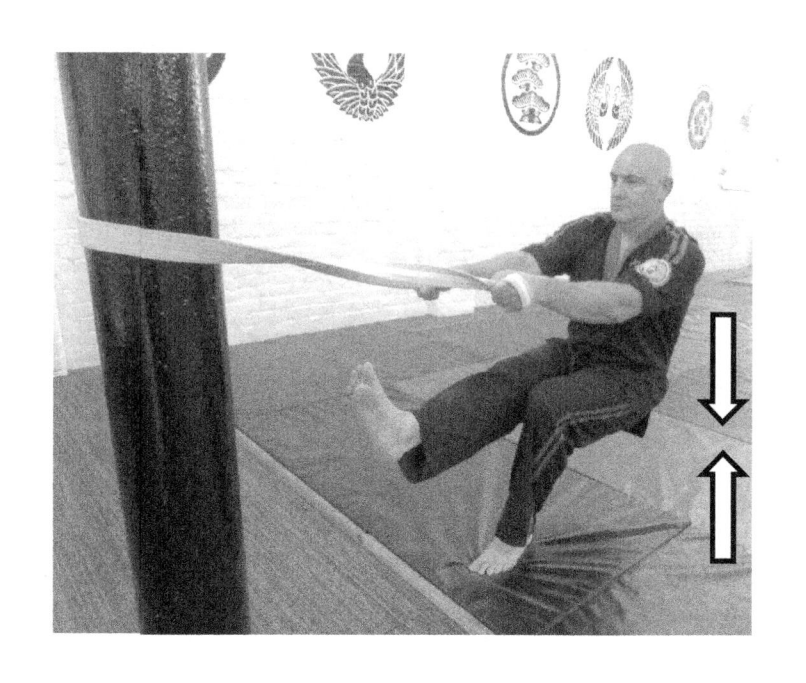

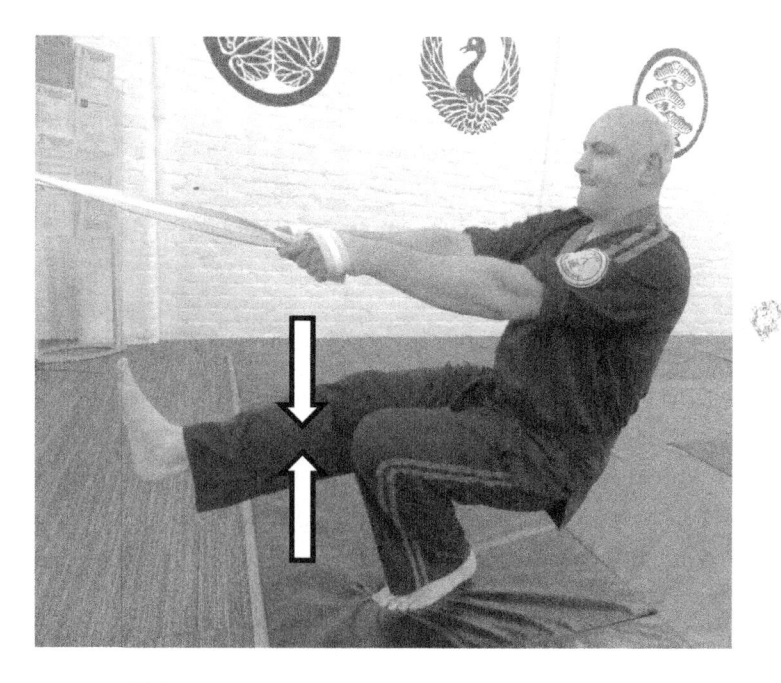

Legs – Belt Squat Hold

Stand evenly on an unfurled martial arts belt with both feet approximately shoulder-width apart. Bend the knees to assume a squat position, making sure to keep your back straight and bend forward only from the hips. Assume a squat position so that your thighs are approximately parallel to the floor. Hold each side of the belt at an appropriate length. Use the force generated by the thighs to try and stand upright while keeping your back straight and hips aligned. The belt secured around the feet will provide an immovable object to perform an isometric exercise.

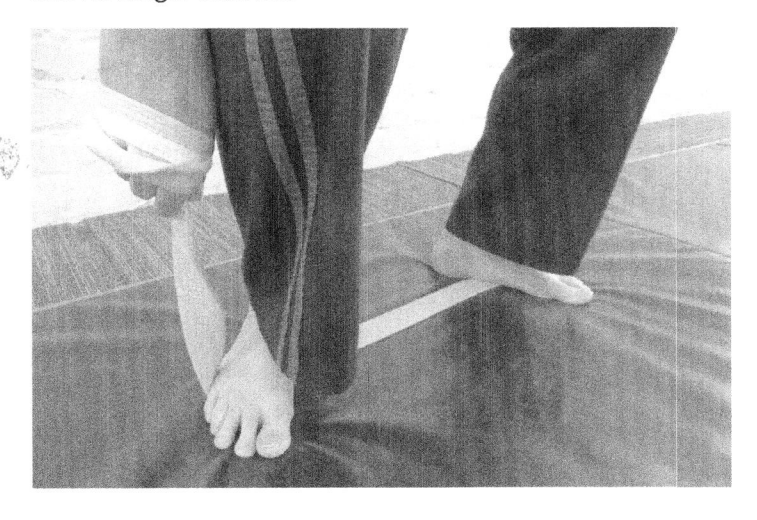

The harder you engage the muscles, the more intense the exercise becomes, so always be sure to exercise at an intensity that best suits your current ability. When you perform an isometric exercise never hold your breath. Always breathe deeply and naturally, which will be about 10 full breaths in and out at a rate of about 1 second per full breath. Perform each exercise for no less than 7 seconds, and no longer than 10.

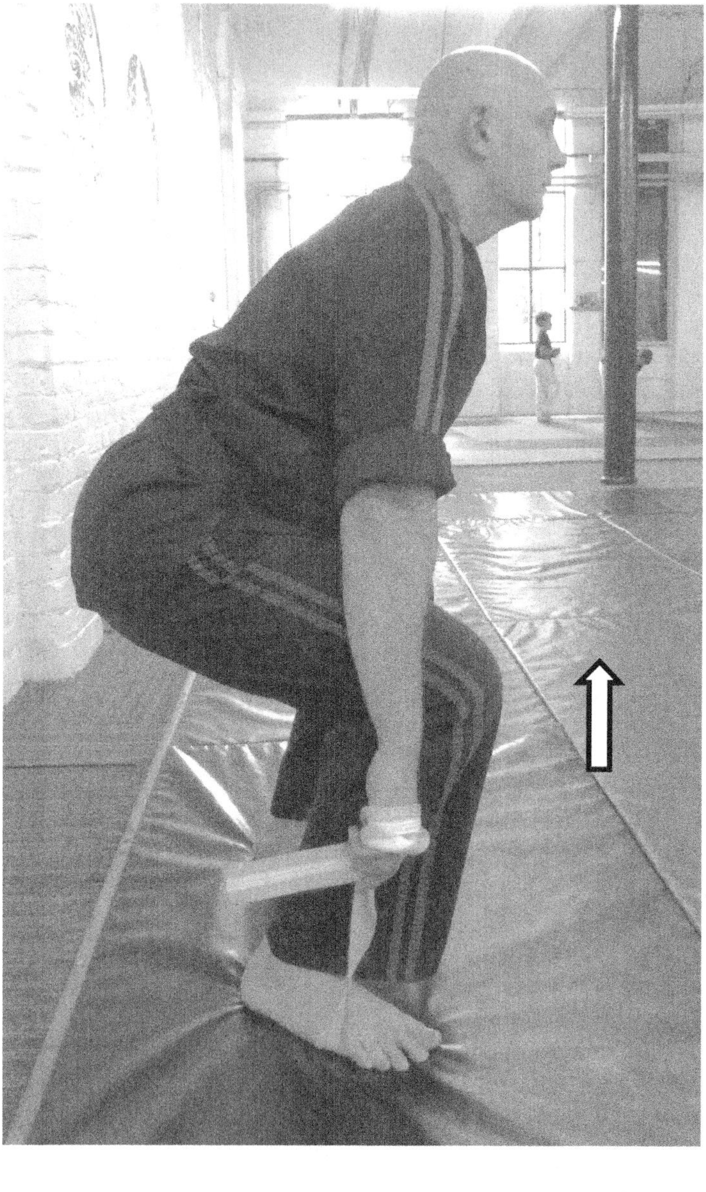

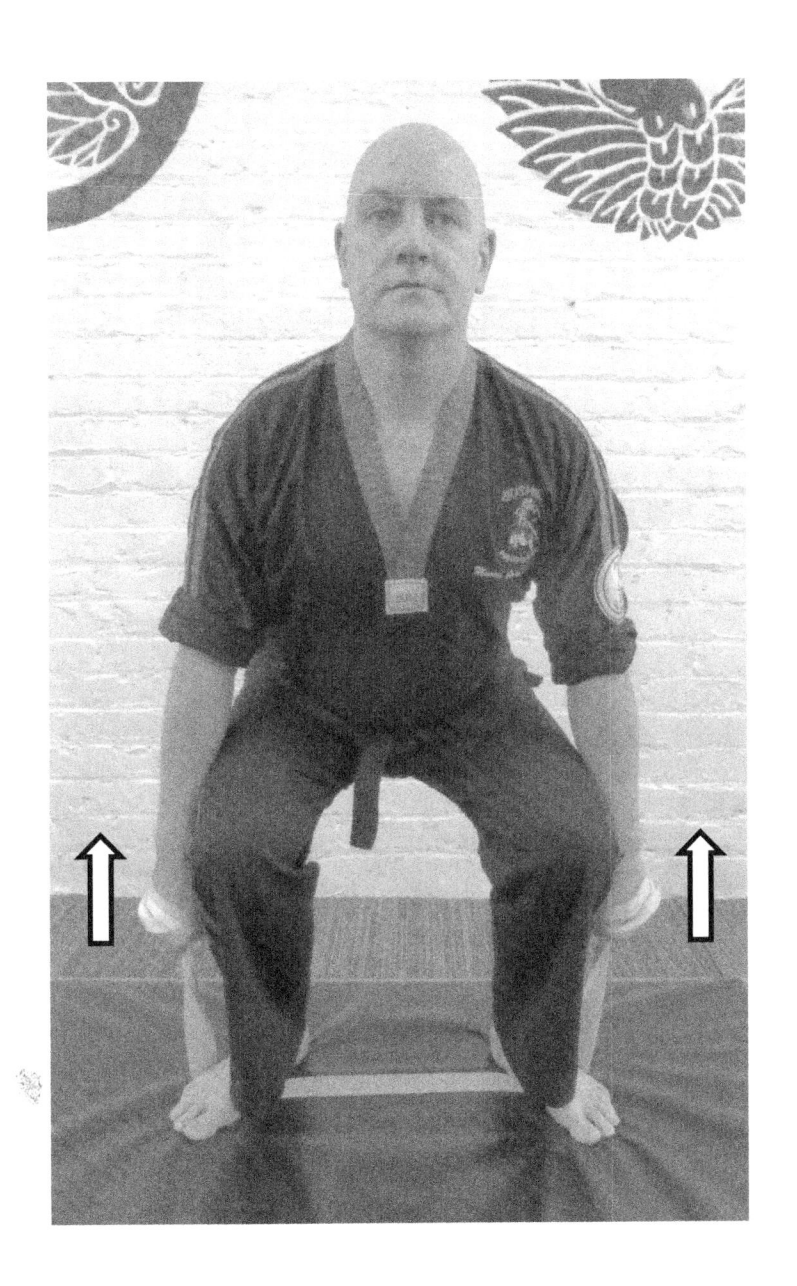

Legs – Wall Squat

Stand with your feet approximately shoulder-width apart approximately one pace away from a wall, pillar, or any other safe, solid object. Lean back against it, and bend the knees into a squat position keeping your back flat and torso engaged against the object. Squat no lower than when the thighs are parallel to the floor. In this position, push backwards and slightly up in a sort of upright leg press by engaging the thigh muscles. When you have generated the desired level of intensity, then perform the isometric exercise. The harder you engage the muscles, the more intense the exercise becomes, so always be sure to exercise at an intensity that best suits your current ability. When you perform an isometric exercise never hold your breath. Always breathe deeply and naturally, which will be about 10 full breaths in and out at a rate of about 1 second per full breath. Perform each exercise for no less than 7 seconds, and no longer than 10.

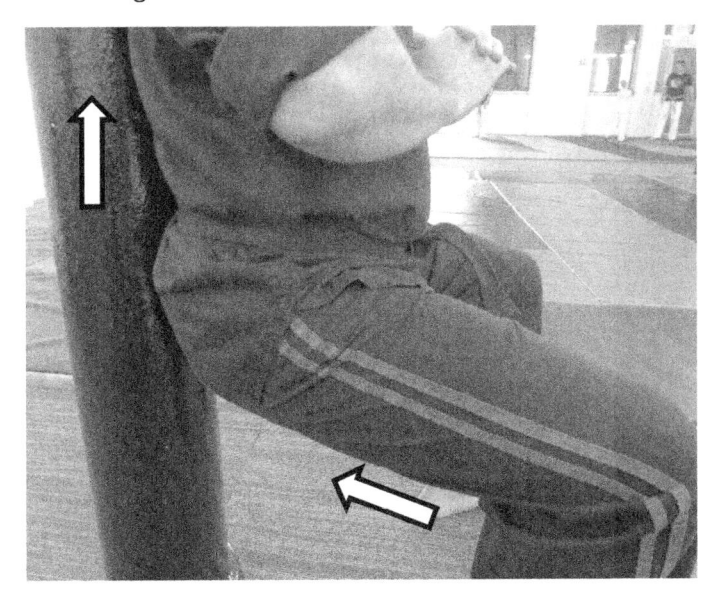

225

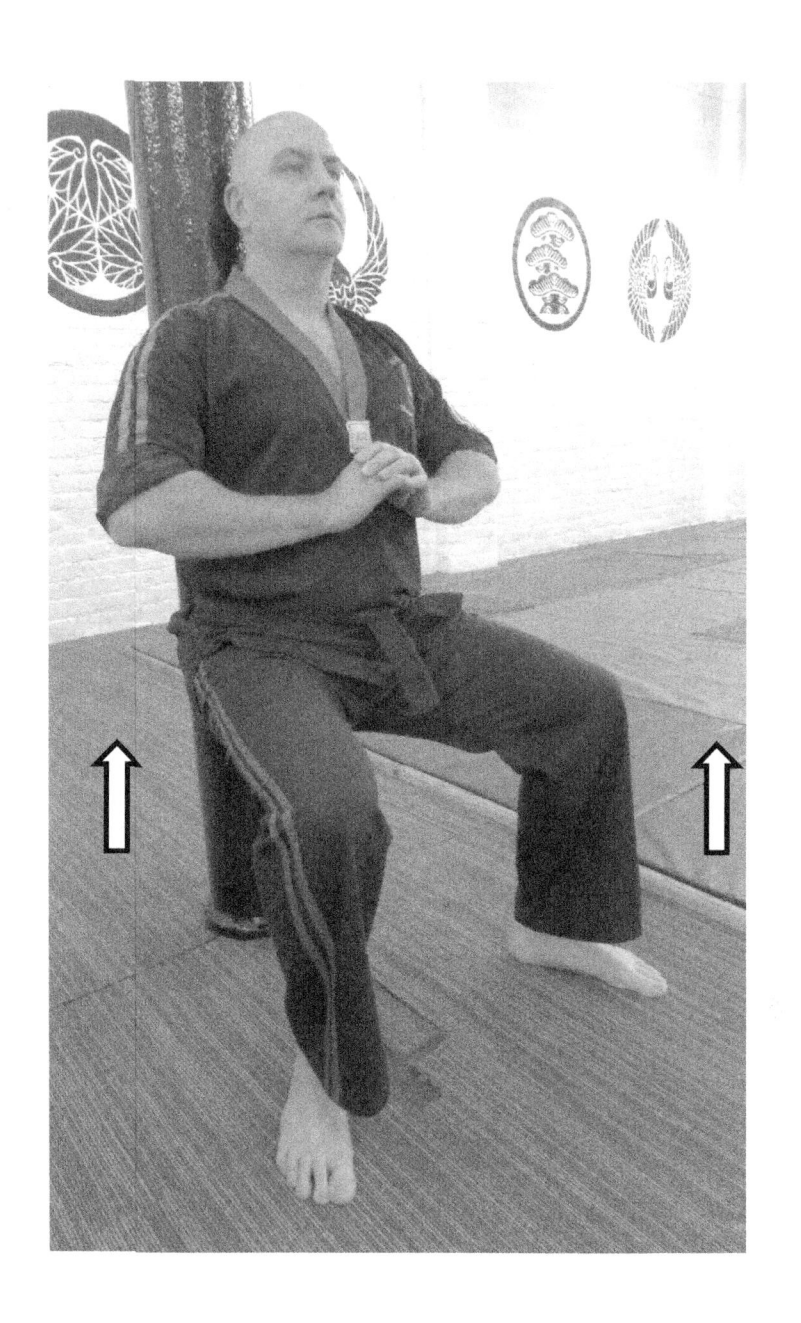

Legs – Partner Shoulder Squat

First, partner with someone of approximately equal weight. The exercising partner stands with their feet approximately shoulder-width apart. The Support partner stands on a chair, bench or any other solid, safe object that allows them to climb onto the exercising partner's shoulders.

Once on the shoulders of the exercising partner, the supporting partner should tuck their feet and legs around the waist and behind the back of the exercising partner. Once there, they should push slightly to support the exercising partner's lower back. The exercising partner should firmly hold the lower legs/knees of the support partner, then slowly descend into a squat position.

Only descend as deep into a squat as is comfortable and safe to do so. Once the desired level has been reached, then the isometric exercise can be performed. Make sure that the lowest point of any squat is when the thighs are approximately parallel to the floor. When one partner has completed the exercise, swap over so that the other partner may do the same.

The harder you engage the muscles, the more intense the exercise becomes, so always be sure to exercise at an intensity that best suits your current ability. When you perform an isometric exercise never hold your breath.

Always breathe deeply and naturally, which will be about 10 full breaths in and out at a rate of about 1 second per full breath. Perform each exercise for no less than 7 seconds, and no longer than 10.

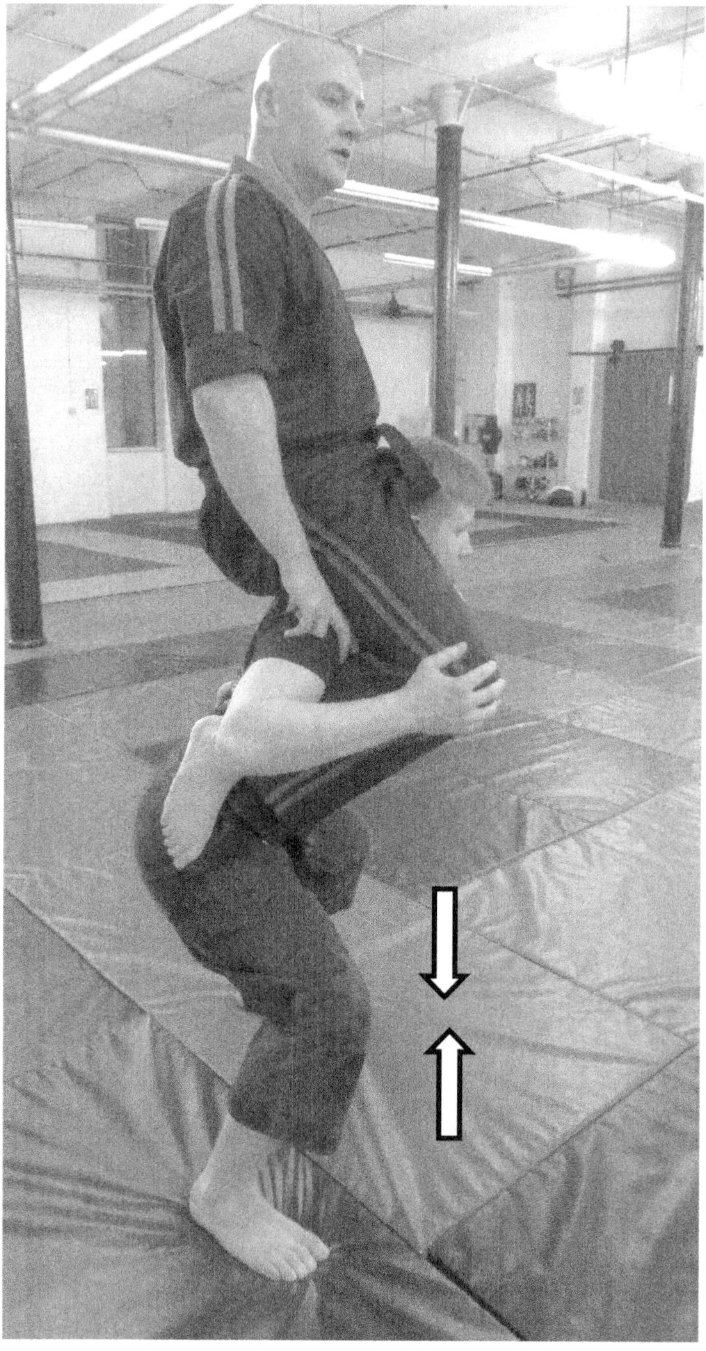

228

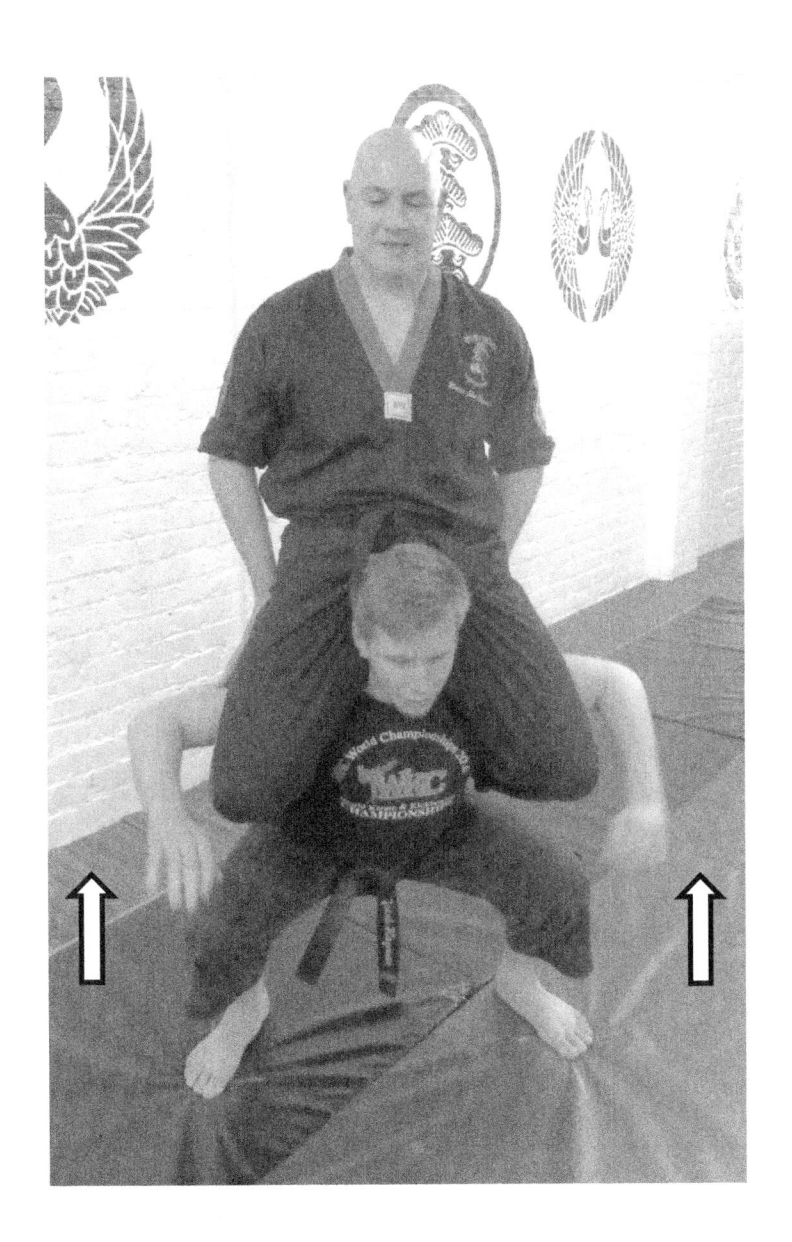

Shoulders – Delta Shoulder Dip Hold

Place both hands on the floor or mat wider than shoulder-width apart.

Make sure the spacing is such that when the arms are bent at the midpoint the elbows will be bent at approximately 90 degrees.

Form a delta 'V' shape with your body between your feet and hands. Your feet should be shoulder-width apart for stability.

Your body should be bent at the waist so that your back is bent only from the hip and remains straight throughout the exercise.

Lower your torso and head towards the mat/floor and stop just short of touching it. This should engage the shoulder muscles. Once in that position, perform the isometric exercise.

The harder you engage the muscles, the more intense the exercise becomes, so always be sure to exercise at an intensity that best suits your current ability. When you perform an isometric exercise never hold your breath.

Always breathe deeply and naturally, which will be about 10 full breaths in and out at a rate of about 1 second per full breath. Perform each exercise for no less than 7 seconds, and no longer than 10.

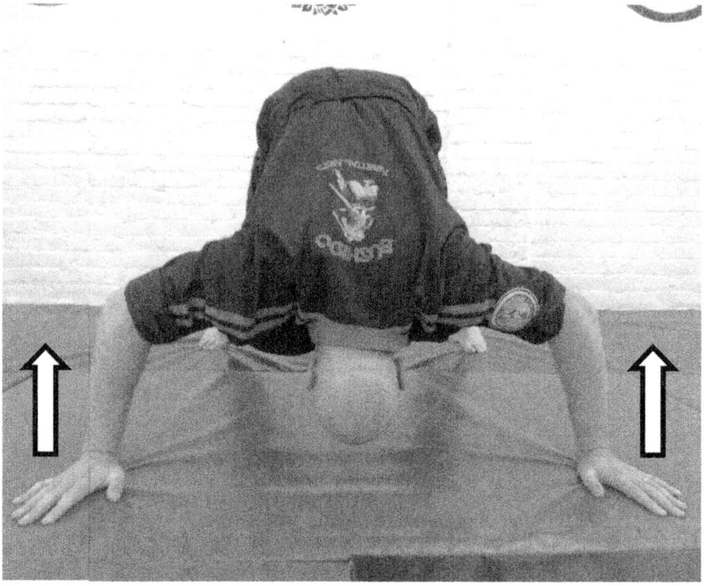

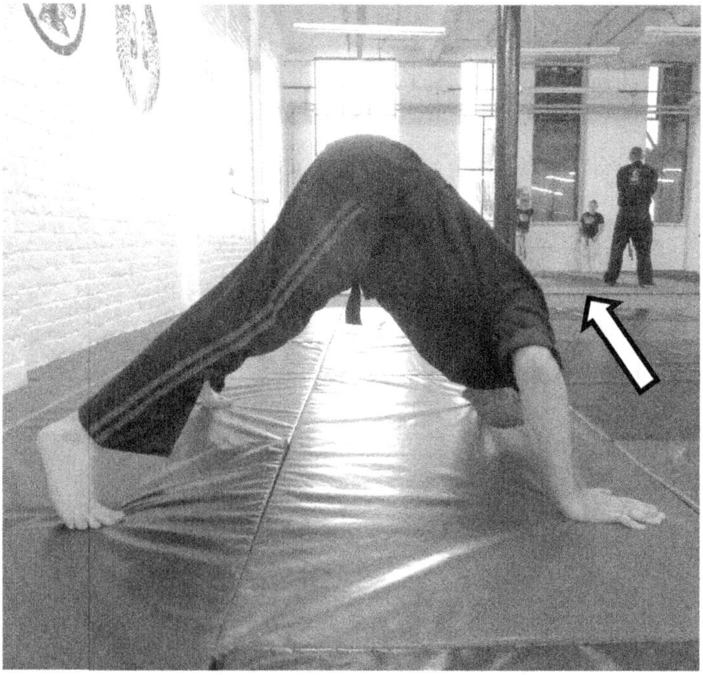

Shoulders – Kneeling Belt Shoulder Press

Kneel on the floor or mat with your legs naturally spaced together in neutral. Place an unfurled martial arts belt evenly under the knees/lower legs so they can secure it when lifted upwards. Hold each of the other ends of the belt and loop it around the hands. Bring both arms up to a position slightly wider than shoulder-width apart and apply force to push upwards using the belt to provide your shoulders with an immovable object. Once you have achieved the target height of the upward press, then apply the desired level of intensity and perform the isometric exercise.

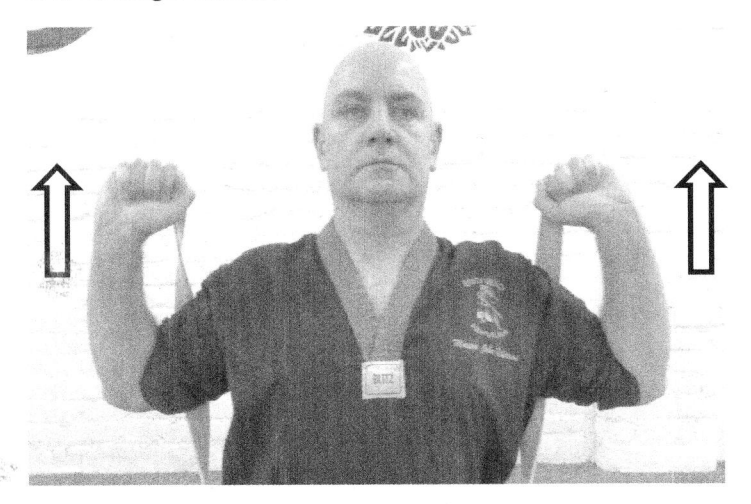

The harder you engage the muscles, the more intense the exercise becomes, so always be sure to exercise at an intensity that best suits your current ability. When you perform an isometric exercise never hold your breath. Always breathe deeply and naturally, which will be about 10 full breaths in and out at a rate of about 1 second per full breath. Perform each exercise for no less than 7 seconds, and no longer than 10.

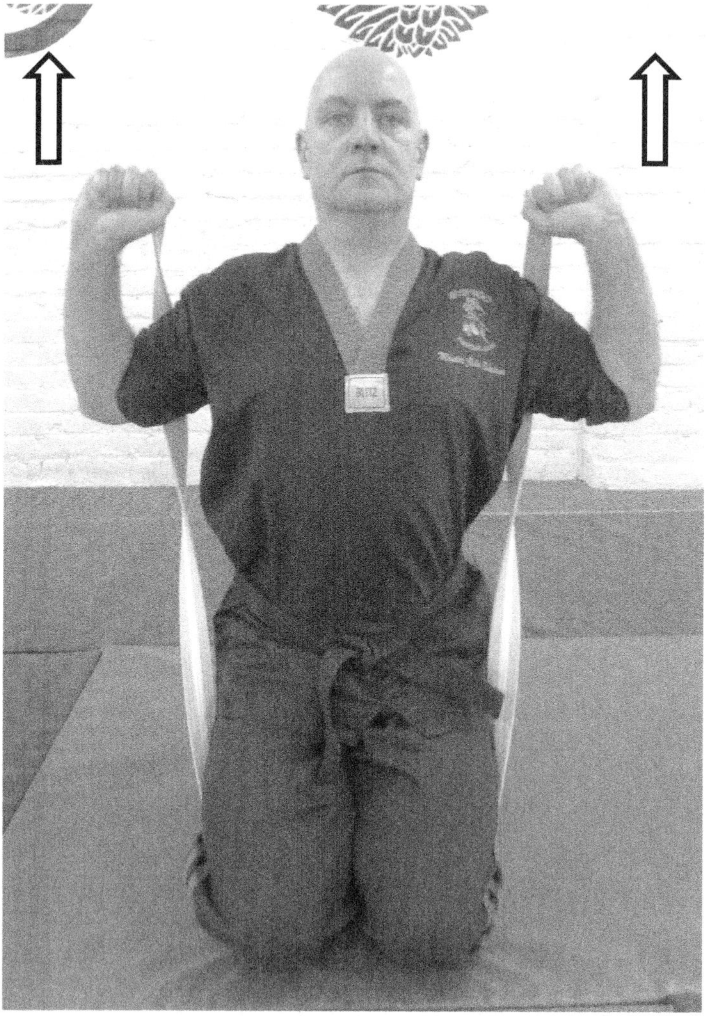

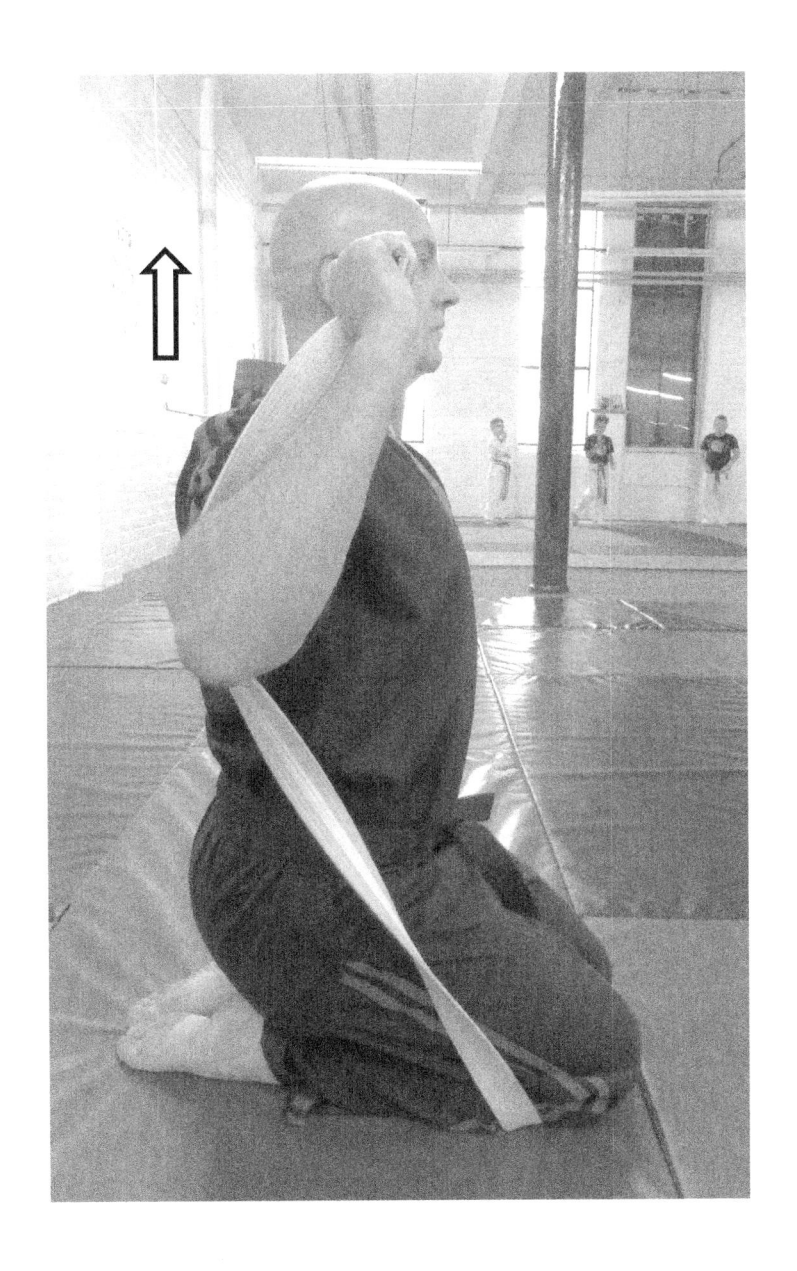

Shoulders – Upright Belt Pull

Stand with your feet approximately shoulder-width apart. Place an unfurled martial arts belt evenly under both feet and hold each of the ends, one in each hand at approximately the point where the stomach meets the chest. Loop the belt around the hands to make it secure. Ensuring that your arms are kept slightly away from the body and keeping the elbows forwards, apply force to lift the immovable belt using your shoulder muscles as the primary driving force. Once you have achieved both the desired position and level of intensity, then perform the isometric exercise.

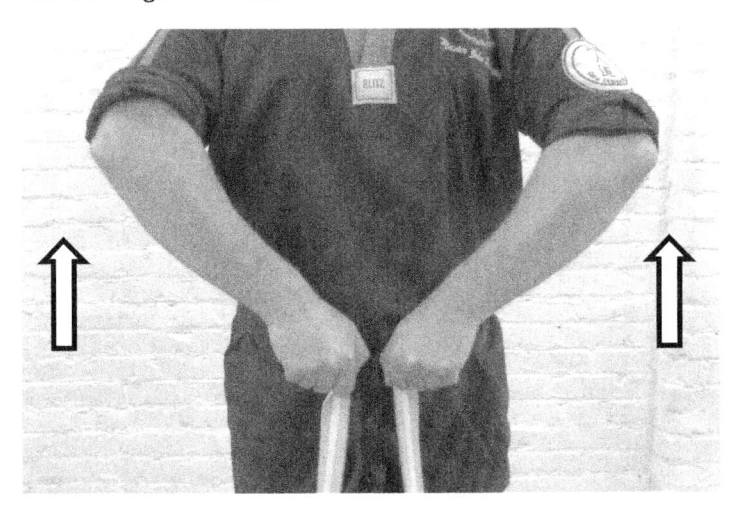

The harder you engage the muscles, the more intense the exercise becomes, so always be sure to exercise at an intensity that best suits your current ability. When you perform an isometric exercise never hold your breath. Always breathe deeply and naturally, which will be about 10 full breaths in and out at a rate of about 1 second per full breath. Perform each exercise for no less than 7 seconds, and no longer than 10.

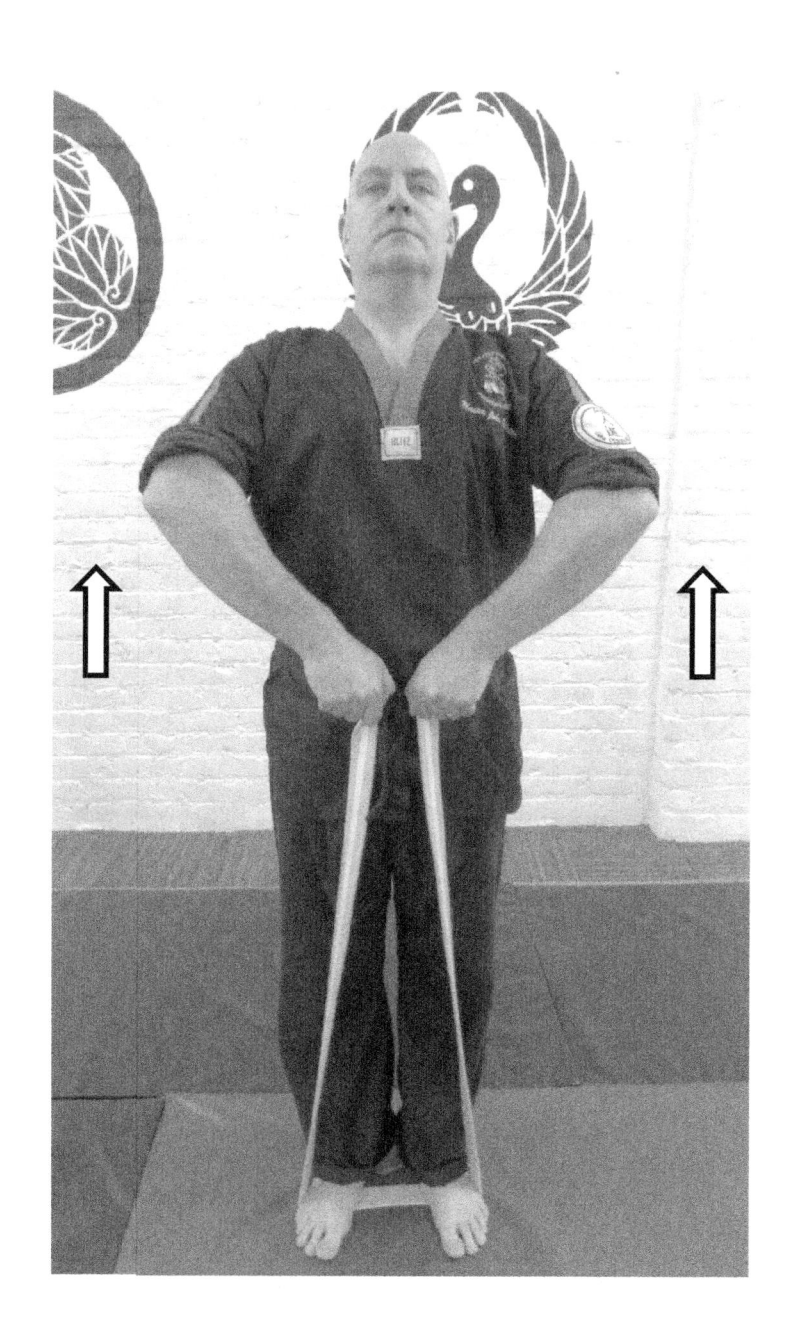

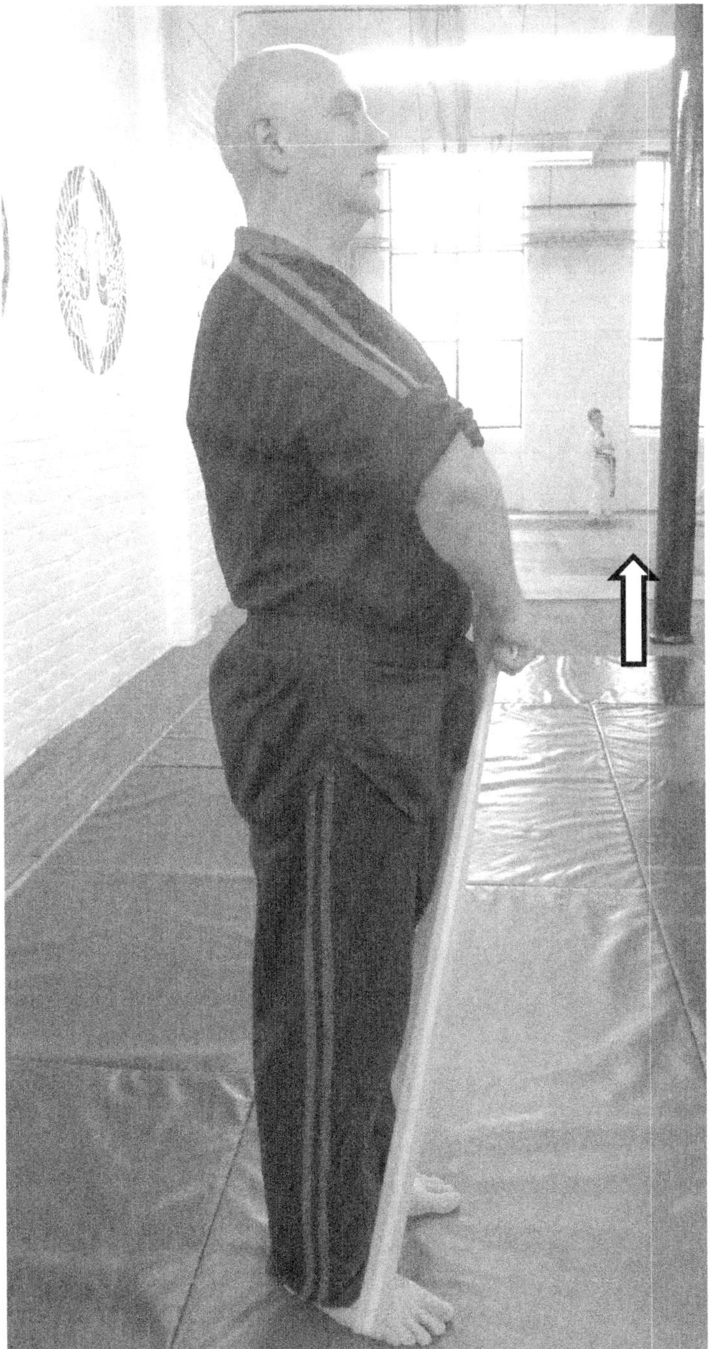

Shoulders
Lateral Raise Belt Pull-Apart Midpoint

Stand with your feet approximately shoulder-width apart. Hold an unfurled martial arts belt evenly in both hands at about waist level in front of you. Loop the loose ends of the belt around the hands. Bend both arms slightly and lock the elbows in that bent position so they do not move during the exercise. Using the shoulder muscles as the primary driving force, attempt to pull the belt apart. Naturally, this is impossible, but it will allow you to exercise the shoulders with an isometric exercise at the desired level of intensity. The harder you engage the muscles, the more intense the exercise becomes, so always be sure to exercise at an intensity that best suits your current ability. When you perform an isometric exercise never hold your breath. Always breathe deeply and naturally, which will be about 10 full breaths in and out at a rate of about 1 second per full breath. Perform each exercise for no less than 7 seconds, and no longer than 10.

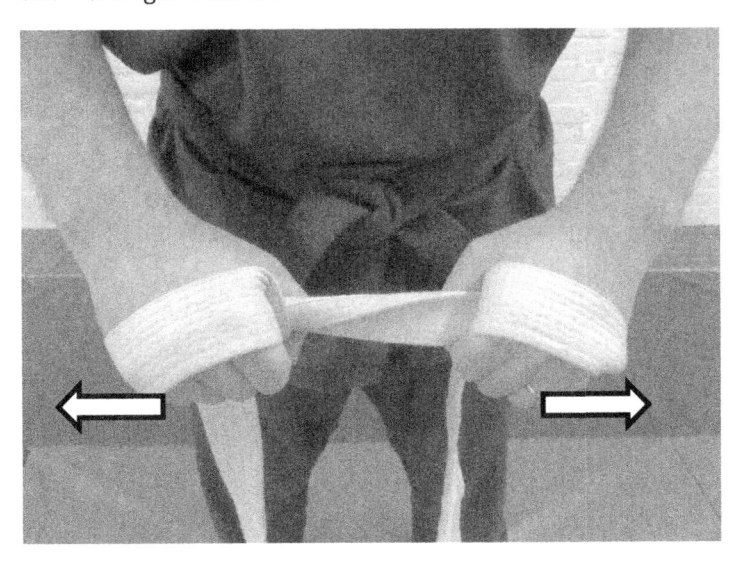

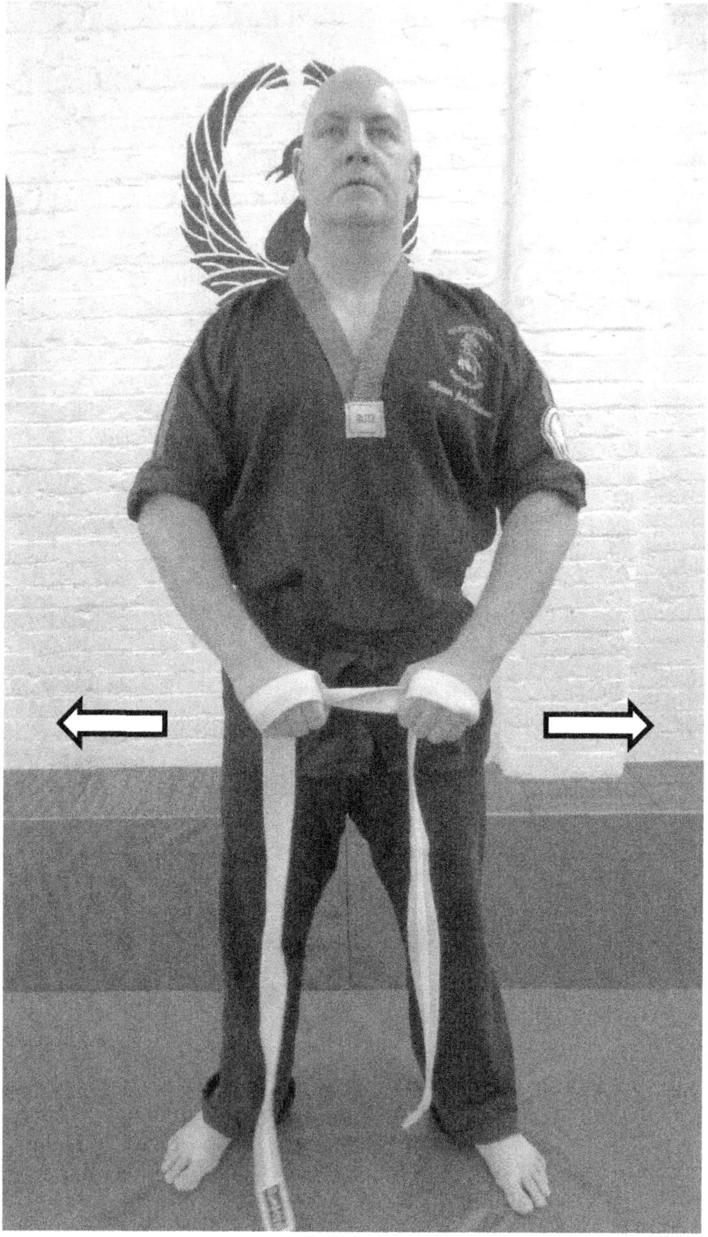

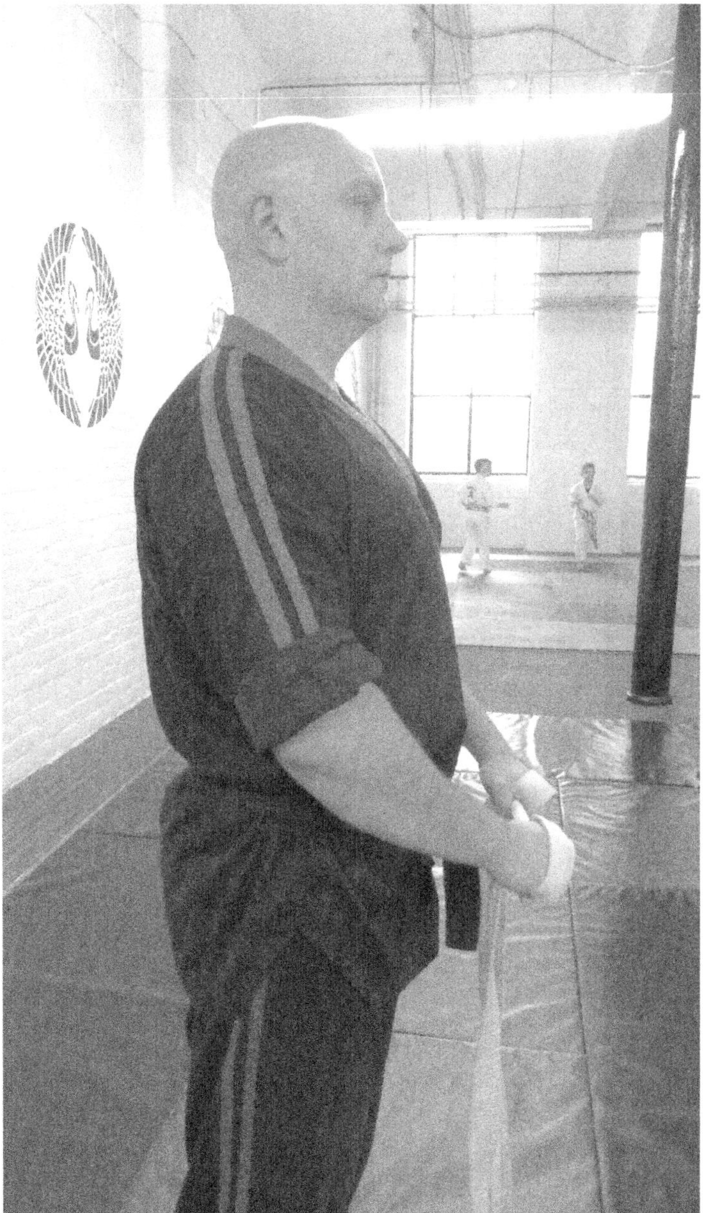

Shoulders
Lateral Raise Belt Pull-Apart - Both Sides

Stand with your feet approximately shoulder-width apart. Hold an unfurled martial arts belt evenly in both hands at about waist level in front of you.

Loop the loose ends of the belt around the hands. Bend both arms slightly and lock the elbows in that bent position so they do not move during the exercise.

Now, lift one arm slightly more to one side of the body like moving the hands on a clock face. Using the shoulder muscles as the primary driving force, attempt to pull the belt apart.

Since this is impossible you can exercise the shoulders with an isometric exercise at the desired level of intensity. Be sure to exercise both sides of the body the same way.

The harder you engage the muscles, the more intense the exercise becomes, so always be sure to exercise at an intensity that best suits your current ability. When you perform an isometric exercise never hold your breath.

Always breathe deeply and naturally, which will be about 10 full breaths in and out at a rate of about 1 second per full breath. Perform each exercise for no less than 7 seconds, and no longer than 10.

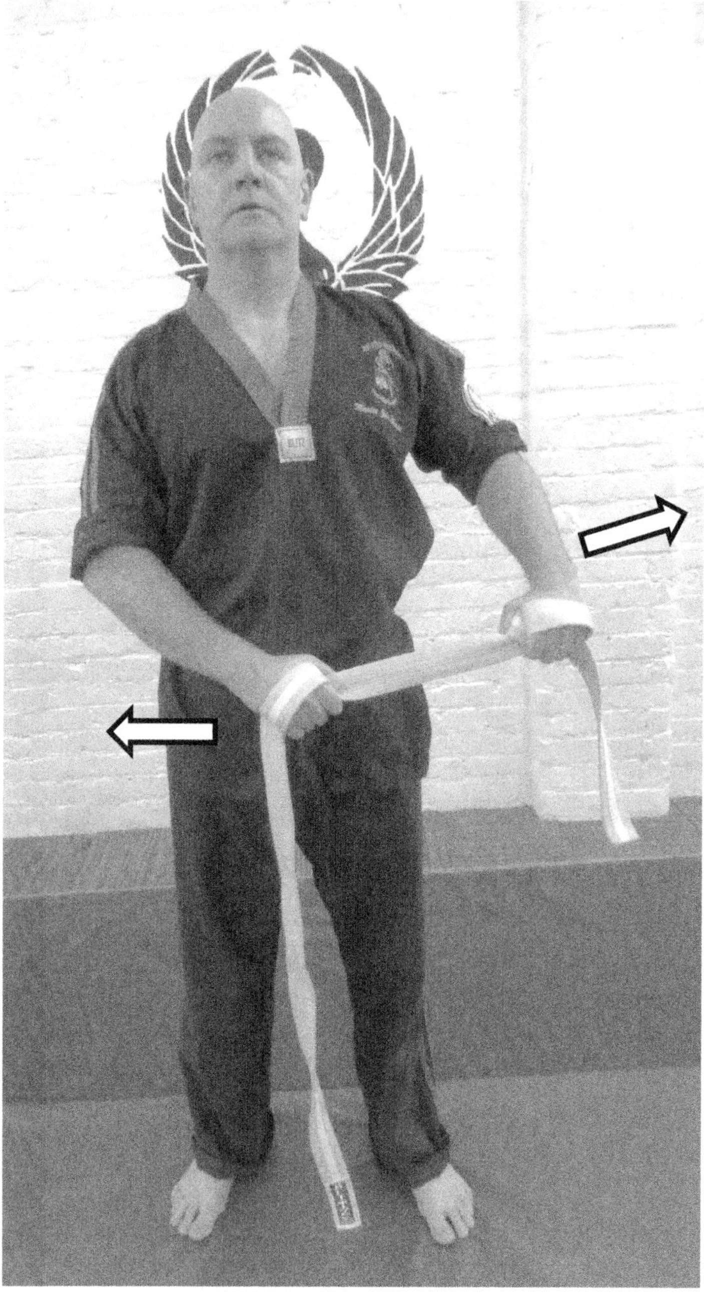

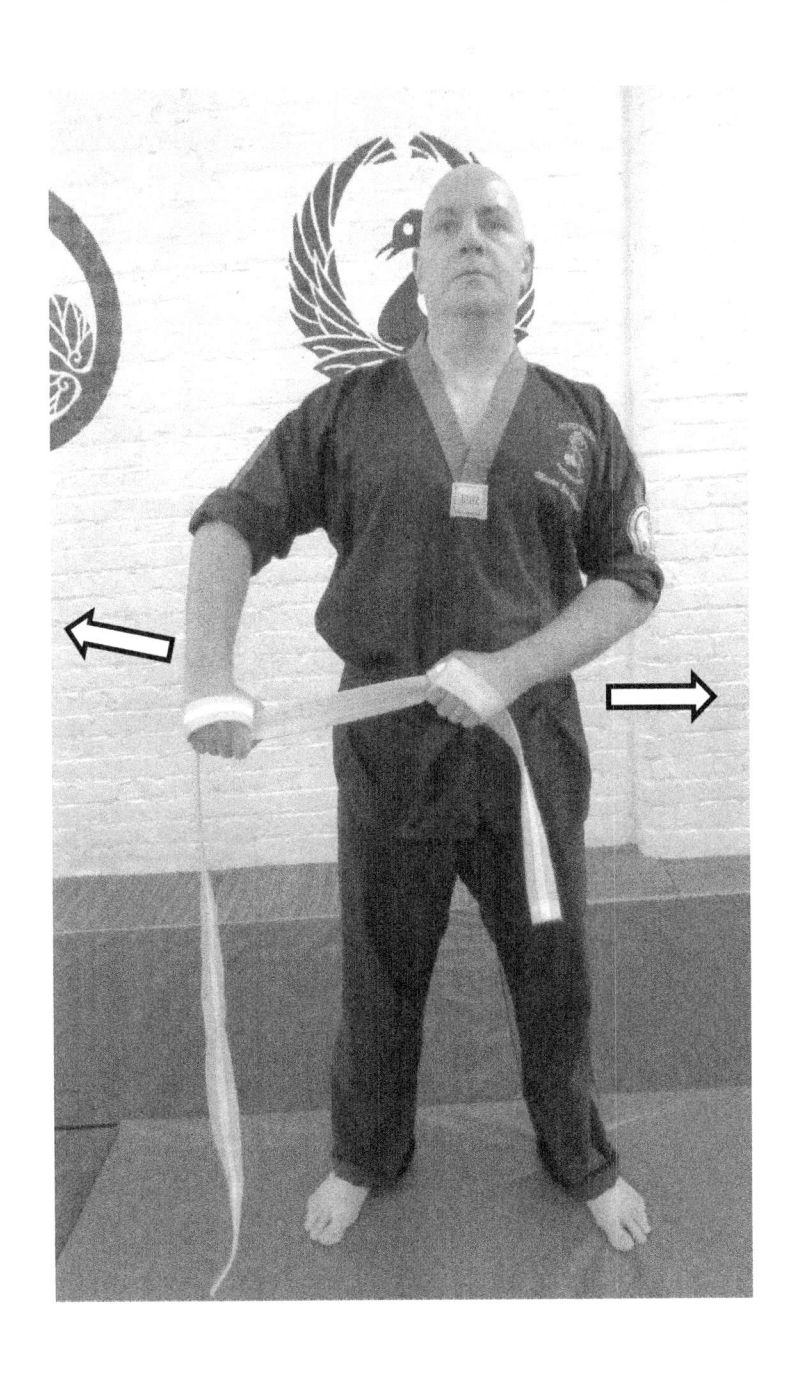

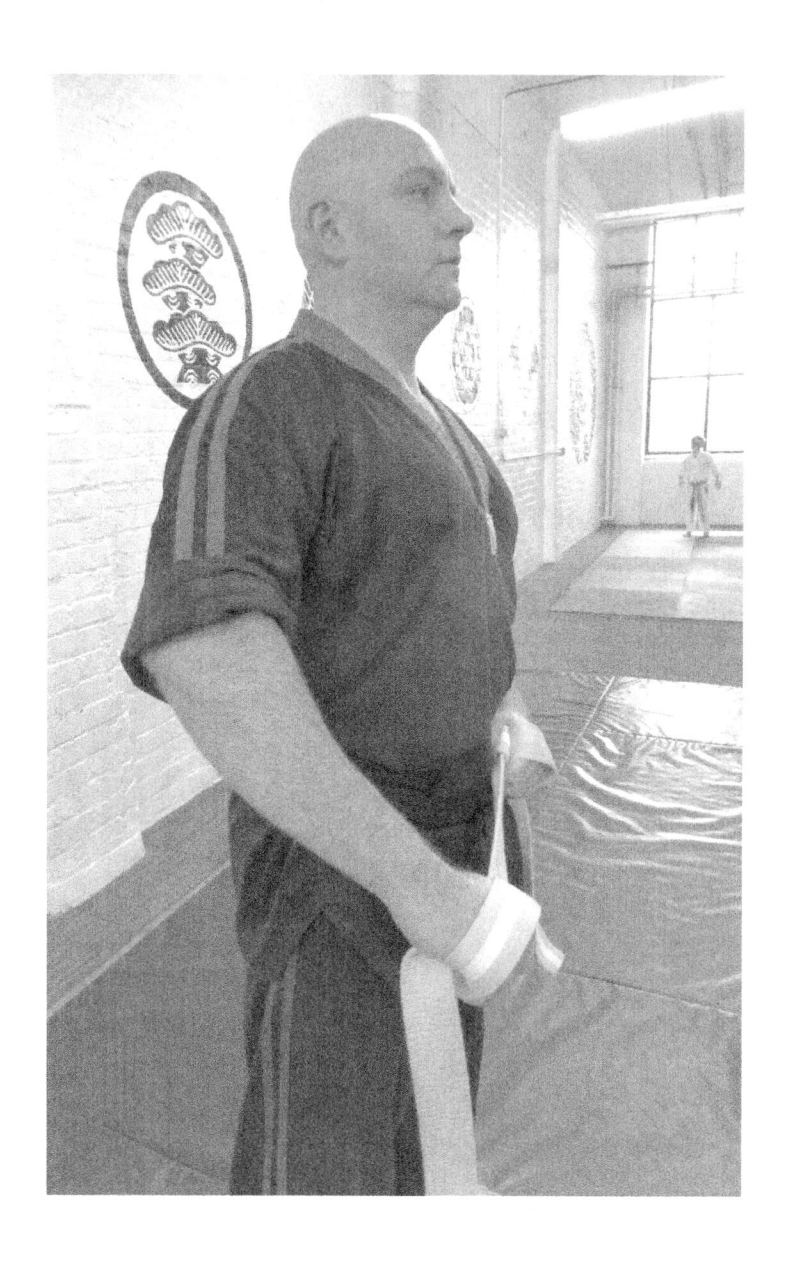

Shoulders – Forward Raise Belt Pull-Apart

Stand with your feet approximately shoulder-width apart. Hold an unfurled martial arts belt evenly in both hands at about waist level in front of you. Loop the loose ends of the belt around the hands. Bent both arms slightly and lock the elbows in that bent position so they do not move during the exercise. Now, lift one arm forward to about chest height, while the other end is secured at waist height by the other hand. Using the front shoulder muscle as the primary driving force, attempt to pull the belt apart. Since this is impossible you can exercise the shoulders with an isometric exercise at the desired level of intensity. Be sure to exercise both sides of the body the same way. The harder you engage the muscles, the more intense the exercise becomes, so always be sure to exercise at an intensity that best suits your current ability. When you perform an isometric exercise never hold your breath. Always breathe deeply and naturally, which will be about 10 full breaths in and out at a rate of about 1 second per full breath. Perform each exercise for no less than 7 seconds, and no longer than 10.

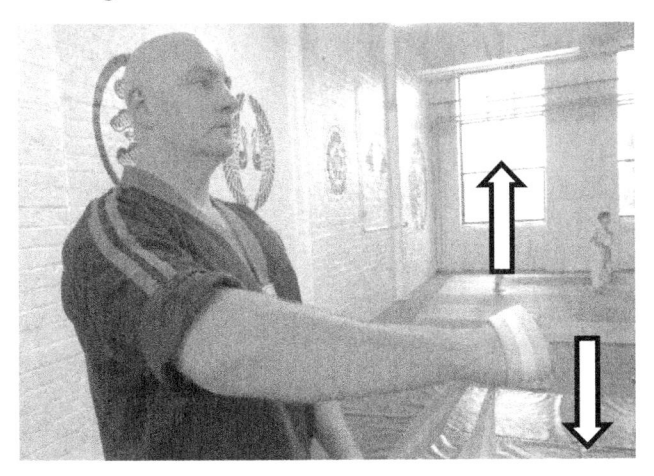

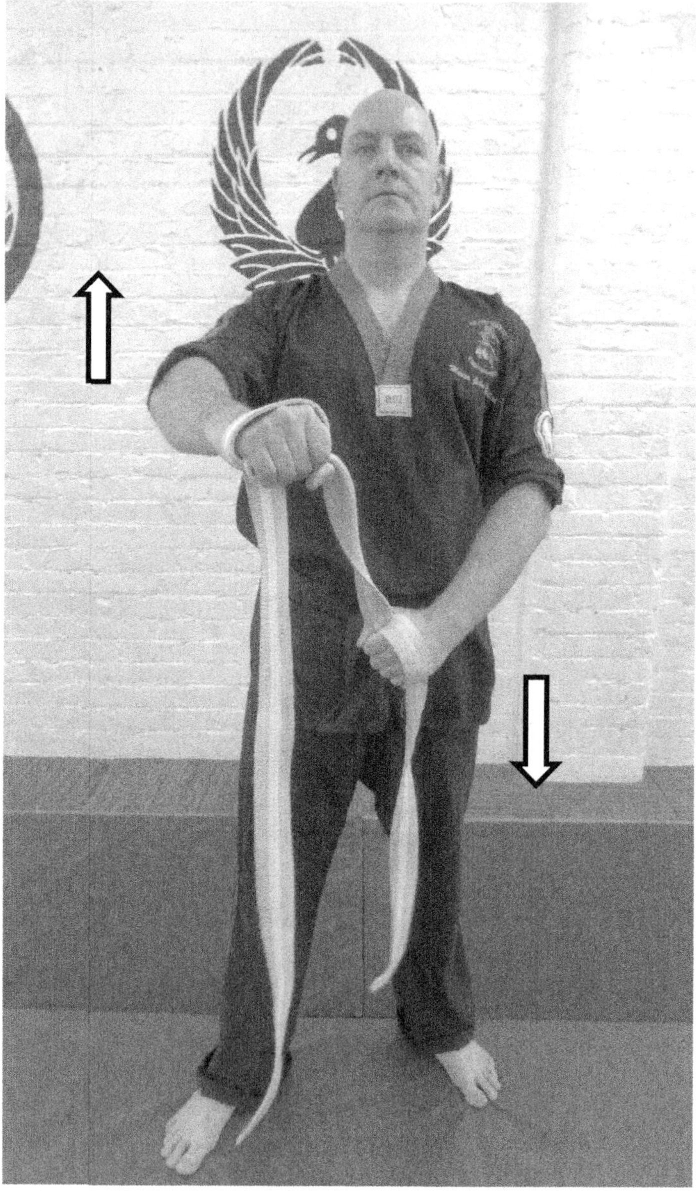

Neck – Forward Belt Head Nod

Stand with your feet approximately shoulder-width apart. Hold an unfurled martial arts belt evenly in both hands. Wrap the midpoint of the belt against the forehead. Both hands should hold the loose ends of the belt at head height above the shoulders. Wrap both ends of the belt around the hands. In this position, gently apply forward and downward pressure to the belt as if performing a head nod that is resisted by the belt. Perform an isometric exercise in this position. Always use caution and never apply too much force or apply force too quickly. If in any doubt do not perform the exercise. The harder you engage the muscles, the more intense the exercise becomes, so always be sure to exercise at an intensity that best suits your current ability. When you perform an isometric exercise never hold your breath. Always breathe deeply and naturally, which will be about 10 full breaths in and out at about 1 second per full breath. Perform each exercise for no less than 7 seconds, and no longer than 10.

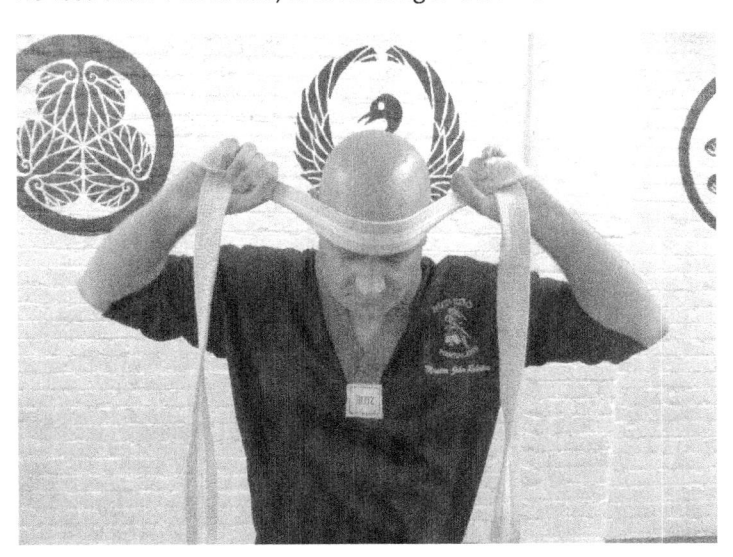

251

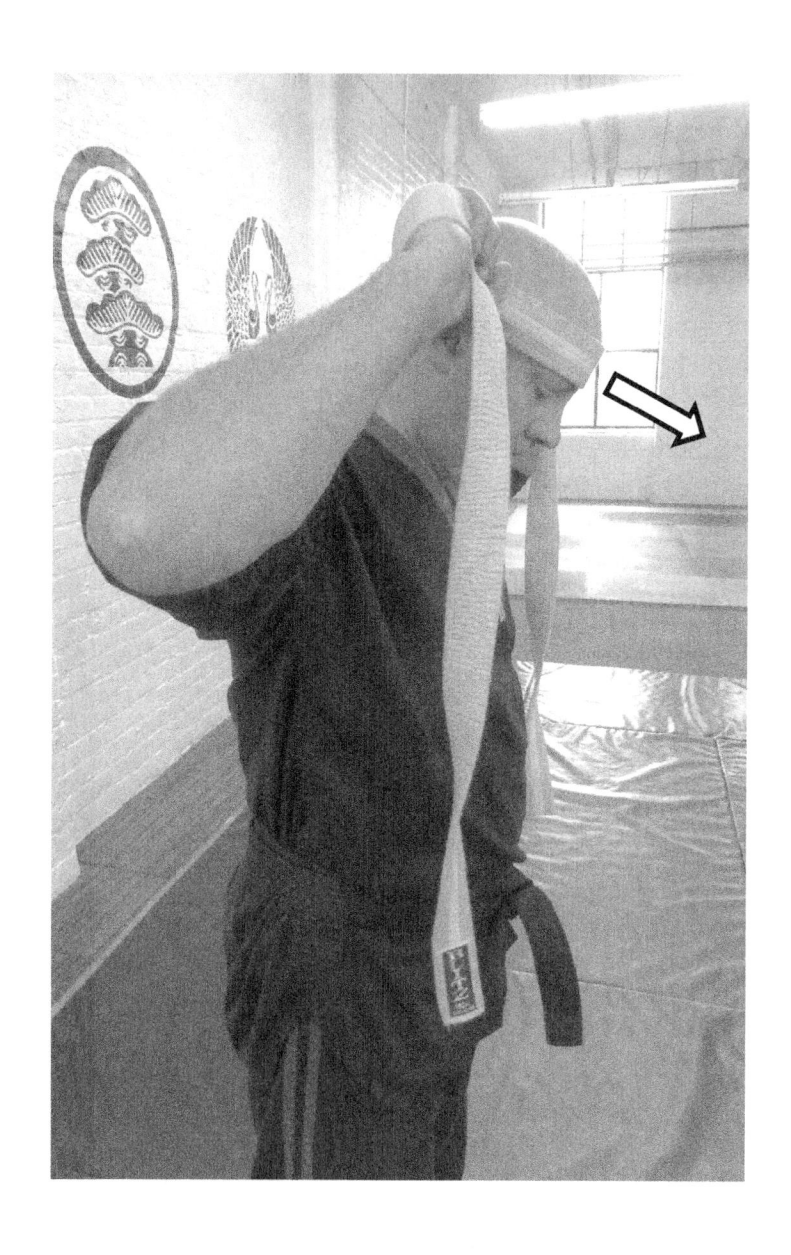

Neck – Backwards Belt Head Nod

Stand with your feet approximately shoulder-width apart. Hold an unfurled martial arts belt evenly in both hands. Wrap the midpoint of the belt against the back of the head. Both hands should hold the loose ends of the belt at head height above the shoulders. Wrap both ends of the belt around the hands. In this position, gently apply backward pressure to the belt as if performing a backward head nod that is resisted by the belt. Perform an isometric exercise in this position. Always use caution and never apply too much force or apply force too quickly. If in any doubt do not perform the exercise. The harder you engage the muscles, the more intense the exercise becomes, so always be sure to exercise at an intensity that best suits your current ability. When you perform an isometric exercise never hold your breath. Always breathe deeply and naturally, which will be about 10 full breaths in and out about 1 second per full breath. Perform each exercise for no less than 7 seconds, and no longer than 10.

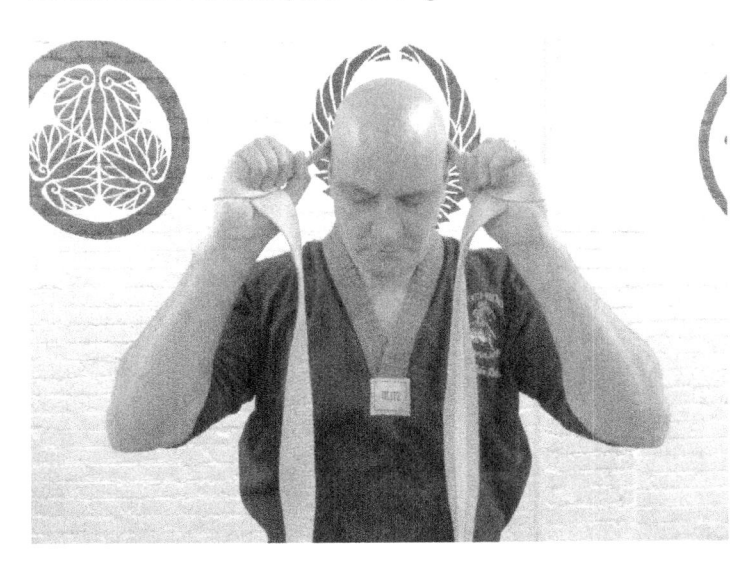

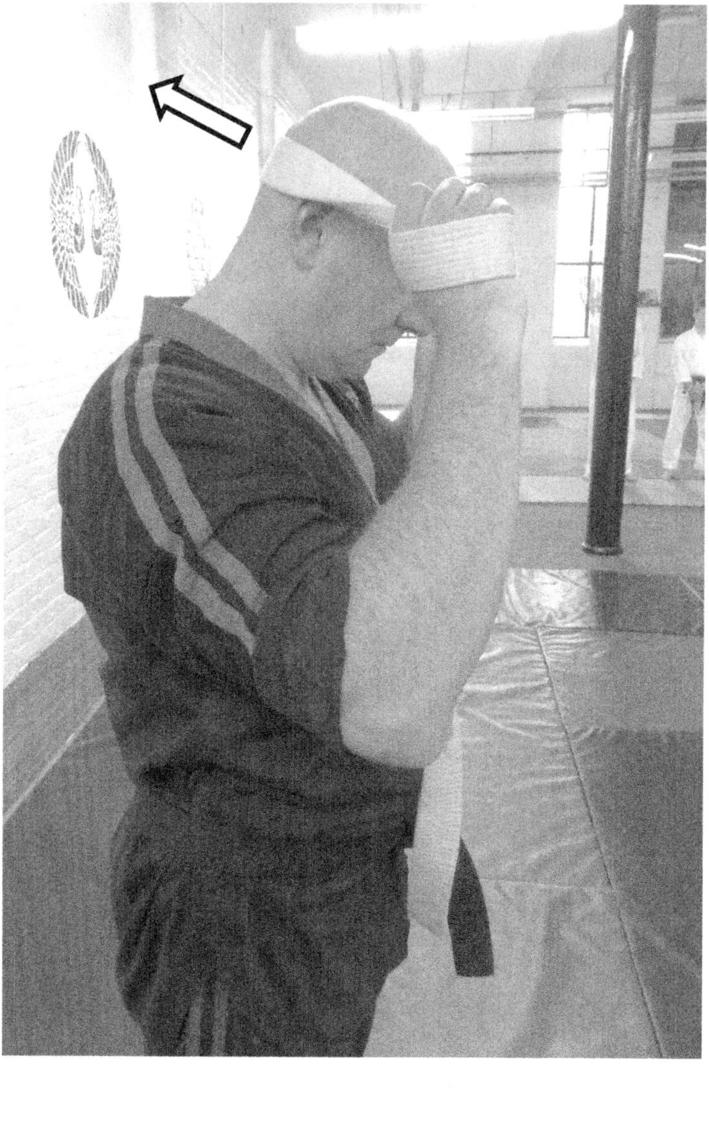

Neck – Side Head Press on Hand

Stand with your feet approximately shoulder-width apart. Lift one arm and place the flat of your hand on the side of your head.

Do not allow your arm to move from this fixed position. gently apply pressure sideward with the head to press against the hand.

Perform an isometric exercise in this position. Always use caution and never apply too much force or apply force too quickly. If in any doubt do not perform the exercise. Be sure to exercise both sides of the neck by changing the hand and arm positions.

The harder you engage the muscles, the more intense the exercise becomes, so always be sure to exercise at an intensity that best suits your current ability. When you perform an isometric exercise never hold your breath.

Always breathe deeply and naturally, which will be about 10 full breaths in and out at a rate of about 1 second per full breath. Perform each exercise for no less than 7 seconds, and no longer than 10.

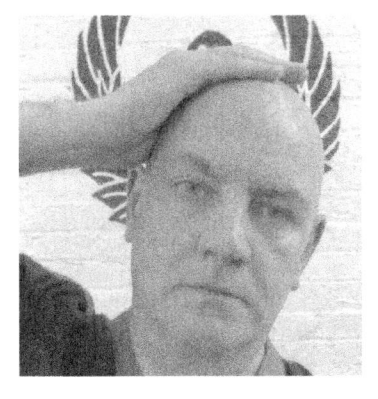

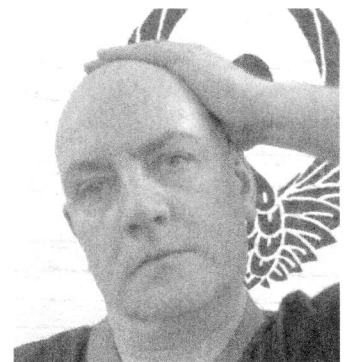

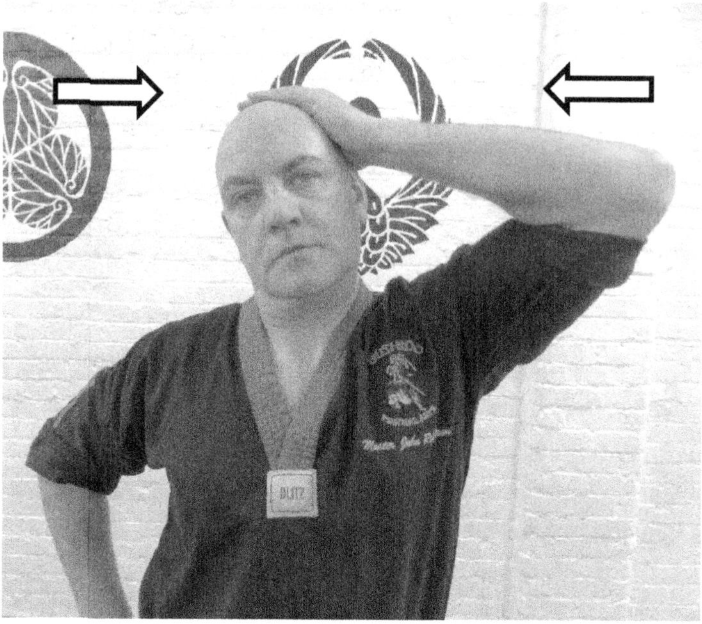

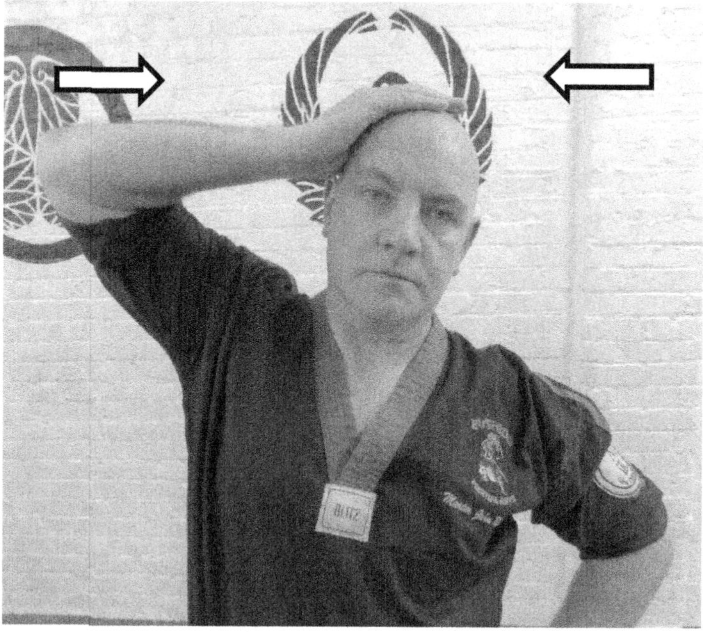

Chapter 8: Conclusion

The practice of any martial art is a life journey. It evolves and develops as the person studying the art grows, develops, and gains wider experience as a human being. The same is true of the practice and incorporation of isometric exercise into your martial art and life in general. No matter which martial art you study and practice, it becomes something that is part of every fibre of who you are as a person. It goes with you like the shadow you cast when walking in the sunlight.

Isometric exercise has much the same effect and impact on virtually everyone who performs it regularly. Once you have experienced your own unique "Eureka" moment; the moment where the proverbial switch is flipped in your mind, then it is impossible to imagine living your life without performing some kind of regular isometric workout session daily.

Isometric exercises are so fast, efficient, and comparatively easy to perform that there is rarely a valid excuse why you did not perform some kind of regular daily exercise routine. I am not suggesting that you mimic the great Bruce Lee and become what many might call exercise-obsessed. Far from it in fact. I am simply suggesting that it is a really good idea to remove isometric exercise from being something one performs during a martial arts training session.

Instead, we suggest that you embrace isometric exercise as a new part of your daily life routine. When it comes to isometric exercise, the effort-to-reward ratio is almost unparalleled. Even if one performs an advanced isometric workout by performing multi-angle exercises for each limb/body part, a total-body exercise routine can still be completed in less than 15-minutes a day – and that is being generous with time.

The 70-Second Difference™ protocol can be performed every day. The 70-Second Difference™ protocol is taken from the book of the same name. It is based on the principle that an isometric workout consisting of 10 x 7-second exercises delivers a comprehensive workout routine for every major muscle group of the body in 70 seconds. Everyone, even on their busiest day, has 70 seconds to spare. Therefore, there are no valid excuses whatsoever why you cannot find the time to exercise regularly.

Ajarn Start Hurst is one of the world's greatest martial artists and he is also an expert exercise instructor. The title, Ajarn, in the Thai language, translates as either "professor" or "teacher." Stuart is both an accredited isometric exercise instructor and also an accredited TRISOmetric™ exercise instructor. The TRISOmetric™ system is an advanced hybrid fusion of isometric and isotonic exercise suitable only for advanced athletes, serious martial arts students, and professional martial arts instructors.

Stuart was the 1st accredited TRISOmetric™ exercise instructor under TWiEA in august 2019 and he now teaches this system as part of his regular coaching and seminar sessions. Master Marc Knowles in Derbyshire, England who kindly modelled for the pictures in this book, is also studying to become a TRISOmetric™ exercise instructor, together with a growing number of instructors from other clubs who are learning how to teach this system. In fact, there are new instructors from all over the world, from the UK to Alaska in the USA, who have been trained by TWiEA. Therefore, if anyone wishes to learn and perform advanced training techniques, there is a method of progression enabling them to do that, and there is an increasing number of coaches who are qualified to teach it.

There are a growing number of serious martial artists or martial arts professionals who are now extending their exercise knowledge base by training with and becoming part of TWiEA, The World Isometric Exercise Association. As TWiEA-approved isometric exercise instructors, it enables them to deliver safe, effective, and enhanced isometric exercise techniques as part of their martial arts coaching sessions, and also as independent exercise coaches and personal trainers.

If you are already a senior-grade martial artist, possibly either a purple or brown belt or higher (or the equivalent depending upon which martial art you practice) then you may wish to explore becoming a TWiEA-approved isometric exercise instructor. For more information about this visit www.TWiEA.com

We sincerely hope that you fully embrace isometric exercise and make the system not simply part of your martial art, but an integral part of your daily life. We wish you every success in your training and life in general. To quote Chapter 64 of the Dao De Jing (that is usually wrongly ascribed to Confucius) when Laozi said, "A journey of a thousand miles begins with a single step" which in Chinese would be 千里之行，始於足下; or Qiānlǐ zhī xíng, shǐyú zú xià. This literally means that "A journey of a thousand Chinese miles starts beneath one's feet" and originated from a famous Chinese proverb. In other words, even the longest and most difficult ventures have a starting point; something which begins with one first step. The same is true when it comes to embracing isometric exercise into your life journey.

www.MajorVision.com

Other books by Brian Sterling-Vete and Helen Renée Wuorio

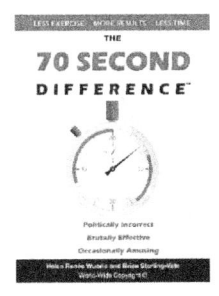

The 70 Second Difference™ - The Politically Incorrect, Occasionally Amusing, and Brutally Effective Guide to Strength, Fitness and Better Health

This book has been approved by **TWiEA** – The World Isometric Exercise Association (www.TWiEA.com).

This is a science-based no-nonsense guide that tells it straight about the most efficient ways to exercise, build muscle, get strong, and how deliberate lifestyle and dietary choices affect you. Lack of time is the main reason why most people don't exercise, however, just 70 seconds a day of focused science-based exercise can solve the problem. Recommended equipment: 2 x Iso-Bows®

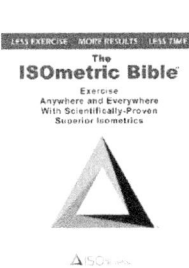

The ISOmetric Bible™ - Exercise Anywhere with Scientifically Proven Isometrics

This book has been approved by **TWiEA** – The World Isometric Exercise Association (www.TWiEA.com).

The ISOmetric Bible™ is a complete, practical, scientific, and user-friendly book. Isometric exercise is proven by science to grow muscle and strength faster and more efficiently than any other exercise system. However, it is also one of the most misunderstood forms of exercise, even by some professionals. No special equipment is needed to get a great total-body workout and this book shows you how to use easy-to-find everyday objects such as walking poles, broom handles, rope, and towels to exercise with. Recommended equipment: 2 x Iso-Bows®, some climbing rope, and a towel.

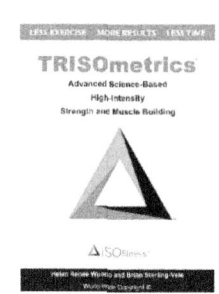

TRISOmetrics™ - Advanced Science-Based High-Intensity Strength and Muscle Building

This book has been approved by **TWiEA** – The World Isometric Exercise Association (www.TWiEA.com).

TRISOmetrics™ is an advanced, science-based high-intensity exercise system that combines 3 scientifically proven exercise techniques into a powerful new exercise system. It can be performed with or without equipment either at home or when travelling, or it can be used as part of a gym-based exercise routine. The system is ideal for people who do not confuse activity with accomplishment. Suggested equipment: 2 x Iso-Bows®, climbing rope and a towel. It can also be performed with the Bullworker®, Steel Bow®, and all gym-based exercise equipment.

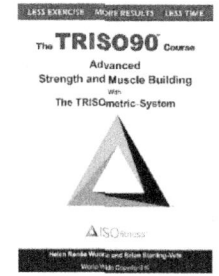

The TRISO90™ Course – Advanced Strength and Muscle Building with The TRISOmetrics™ System

This book has been approved by **TWiEA** – The World Isometric Exercise Association (www.TWiEA.com).

The TRISO90™ Course is a 500+ page 90-day/12-week step-by-step highly advanced bodybuilding/shaping and strength-training exercise course based on the TRISOmetrics™ exercise system. The system consists of three proven science-based exercise principles which when combined, form this highly advanced high-intensity exercise technique, with or without equipment. Suggested equipment: 2 x Iso-Bows®, dipping handles, some climbing rope, and a towel.

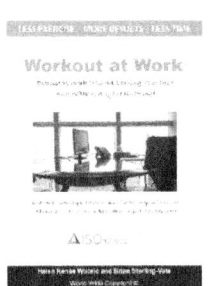

Workout at Work™ - Exercise at Work Without Anyone Even Knowing What You're Doing!

This book has been approved by **TWiEA** – The World Isometric Exercise Association (www.TWiEA.com).

Time is the #1 reason why people do not exercise. The average person spends over 10 years of their life at a desk! With proven isometric exercise, you can exercise effectively at work without ever leaving your desk. Perform just one simple 7-second high-intensity exercise every 30 minutes, and at the end of a 9-hour working day, you will have completed a powerful total-body 18-20 exercise. Your boss will not complain either because in exchange for just 126 seconds of time off work you will be up to 30% more efficient at your job. Recommended equipment: 2 x Iso-Bows®

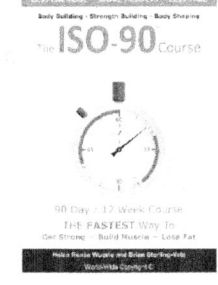

The ISO90™ Course – The 12-Week/90-Day Shape-up and Get Strong Course

This book has been approved by **TWiEA** – The World Isometric Exercise Association (www.TWiEA.com).

The ISO90™ Course is a complete step-by-step 90-day/12-week isometric body shaping, bodybuilding, and strength-building course ideal for both beginners and advanced trainers. Your natural Adaptive Response™ mechanism means that whatever intensity you apply at whatever level you are, gives everyone roughly the same percentage of improvement. Required equipment: 2 x Iso-Bows®

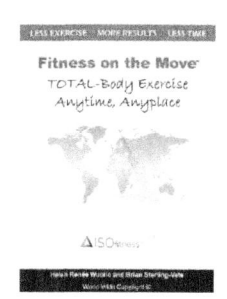

Fitness on the Move™ - Enjoy Gym-Quality Workout Sessions ANYWHERE!

This book has been approved by **TWiEA** – The World Isometric Exercise Association (www.TWiEA.com).

This book lists practical exercises that can be performed while travelling as passengers in cars, on trains, in airline seats, on mountainsides, and beaches etc. A total-body workout can be performed in the smallest space humanly possible thanks to our Zero Footprint Workout™ concept. If there is enough space to either sit down and/or stand upright, then you can perform exercise! Required equipment: 2 x Iso-Bows®

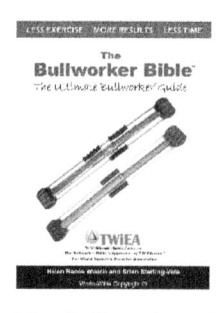

The Bullworker Bible™ The Ultimate Science-Based Guide to The Classic Personal Multi-Gym

This book has been approved by **TWiEA** – The World Isometric Exercise Association (www.TWiEA.com) and the makers of The Bullworker.

The Bullworker Bible™ is THE resource guide for all Bullworker® users and is the companion book to The Bullworker 90™ Course. It is complete, science-based, and user-friendly showing how it should be used to deliver maximum results with information about repetition-compression and speed, breathing, how the laws of physics apply, and correct biomechanics. It is also essential for users of the Steel Bow®, the X5, Bully Extreme, ISO 7x, and the X7. Required: Bullworker® Classic, or similar. Recommended equipment: Steel Bow®, 2 x Iso-Bows®.

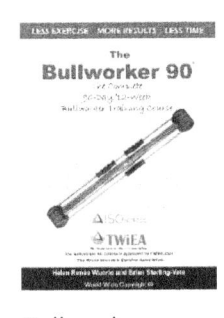

The Bullworker 90™ Course – The Ultimate Science-Based 12-Week/90-Day Get strong and Grow Muscle Course Using the Classic Personal Multi-Gym

This book has been approved by **TWiEA** – The World Isometric Exercise Association (www.TWiEA.com) and the makers of The Bullworker.

The Bullworker 90™ Course is a 90-day/12-week step-by-step course for all Bullworker® users and is the companion book to The Bullworker Bible™. Each week has a detailed note section, so you know exactly what to do and when to do it. It can be used with the Bullworker® Classic, the Steel Bow®, the X5, the Bully Extreme, the ISO 7x, and the X7. The course contains alternative/extra exercises using the Iso-Bow® and the Bow Extension®. Required equipment: Bullworker® Classic, or similar. Recommended equipment: Steel Bow®, Bow Extension® kit, 2 x Iso-Bows®.

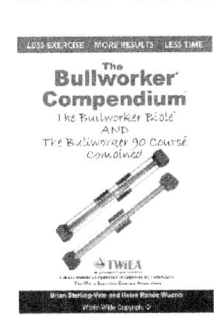

The Bullworker Compendium™ - The Bullworker Bible™ and The Bullworker 90™ Course Combined

This book has been approved by **TWiEA** – The World Isometric Exercise Association (www.TWiEA.com) and the makers of The Bullworker.

The Bullworker Compendium™ is the combination of both The Bullworker Bible™ and The Bullworker 90™ Course in a single huge book. To save printing costs the only thing we have eliminated are duplicated sections, everything else remains the same. This way we can offer both books in one for less than the combined price of the two other books. It starts with The Bullworker Bible™ and progresses seamlessly into The Bullworker 90™ Course.

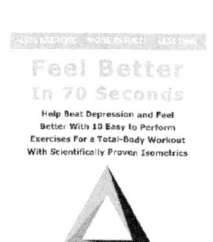

Feel Better In 70 Seconds™

Help Beat Depression and Feel Better With 10 Easy to Perform Exercises For a Total-Body Workout With Scientifically Proven Isometrics

This book has been approved by TWiEA – The World Isometric Exercise Association (www.TWiEA.com). Isolation, depression loneliness, anxiety, and stress are just a few of the serious mental health issues that millions of us can suffer from during our life. Research shows that exercise can help to beat depression and that exercise can be equal to or often better than medication. How can you exercise if you have little or no money, space, motivation, and no idea about exercise? The 70 Second Difference™ is a protocol based upon the premise that 70 seconds of consecutive exercise is needed to perform a 10-exercise total-body workout routine using the scientifically proven isometric exercise system. There is no exercise system we know of that is faster, more effective, and easier to perform.

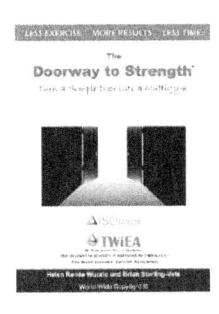

The Doorway to Strength™ - Turn a Door into a Strength-Building Multigym

This book has been approved by **TWiEA** – The World Isometric Exercise Association (www.TWiEA.com).

The Doorway to Strength™ shows how a simple door, doorway, and doorframe can be used to create a multi-gym of exercises using the amazing Iso-Bow® exerciser. It demonstrates how to perform a host of powerful and effective isometric exercises such as the door leg press and shoulder power push, together with many other exercises to work all the major body parts. Required: 2 x Iso-Bows®, a solid door and frame, and a door wedge/stop.

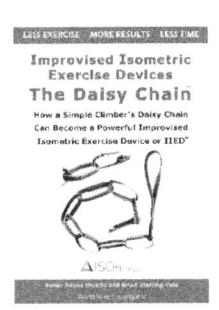

Improvised Isometric Exercise Devices - The Daisy Chain - How a Simple Climber's Daisy Chain Can Become a Powerful Improvised Isometric Exercise Device or IIED

This book has been approved by TWiEA – The World Isometric Exercise Association (www.TWiEA.com).

Improvised Isometric Exercise Devices or IIEDs come in all shapes and sizes and are only limited by your imagination and knowledge of good biomechanics. Basic climbing equipment can also become extremely powerful IIEDs and is both expensive and non-proprietary. One of the most effective is the versatile daisy chain. This is a valuable resource of improvised, practical isometric exercises that can be performed as well as how to safely extend them.

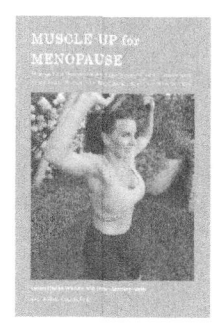

Muscle-up For Menopause

This book has been approved by TWiEA – The World Isometric Exercise Association (www.TWiEA.com).

Menopause can be a devastating rollercoaster ride with many disturbing physical and emotional effects which every woman must face. Since it cannot be avoided, then the best way to approach it is to take control of every element that is within your power to do so. Brief yet intense exercise sessions that place the minimum demand on your ability to recover combined with a high-protein plant-based diet can make all the difference between making life easier or harder as you approach, endure, and emerge from menopause. The exercise course can be performed with no equipment, or with the recommended pair of Iso-Bows®, and/or Improvised Isometric Exercise Devices or IIEDs that are readily available to most people.

Improvised Isometric Exercise Devices - The Climber's Sling - How a Simple Climber's Sling Can Become a Powerful Improvised Isometric Exercise Device or IIED

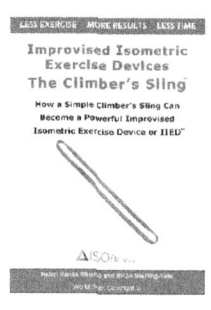

This book has been approved by TWiEA – The World Isometric Exercise Association (www.TWiEA.com).

Improvised Isometric Exercise Devices or IIEDs come in all shapes and sizes and are only limited by your imagination and knowledge of good biomechanics. Basic climbing equipment can also become extremely powerful IIEDs and is both expensive and non-proprietary. One of the most effective is the versatile Climber's sling. This is a valuable resource of improvised, practical isometric exercises that can be performed as well as how to safely extend them.

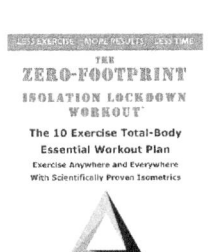

The Zero-Footprint Isolation Lockdown Workout
The 10 Exercise Total-Body Essential Workout Plan Exercise Anywhere and Everywhere With Scientifically Proven Isometrics

This book has been approved by TWiEA – The World Isometric Exercise Association (www.TWiEA.com).

In 2020, the world changed forever due to the COVID-19 global pandemic and gyms are typically some of the unhealthiest of places when it comes to virus and disease transmissions. Millions of people who love to exercise were suddenly forced to learn how to exercise at home, sometimes in very confined spaces. The Zero-Footprint Isolation Lockdown Workout™ delivers the 10 essential total-body isometric exercises that can be performed in the smallest of spaces. If you can stand and sit, then you can perform a powerful workout routine in as little as 70 seconds a day! NOTE: This is a variation of The 70 Second Difference™ workout.

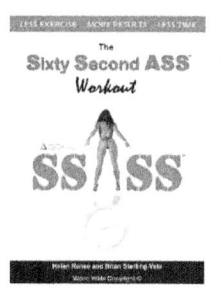

The Sixty Second ASS Workout™ - The Ultimate 60-Second Workout to Shape, Tone, Lift and Give You the Backside You've Always Wanted

This book has been approved by **TWiEA** – The World Isometric Exercise Association (www.TWiEA.com).

The Sixty Second ASS Workout™, or SSASS™ workout, is the fastest and most effective "ass" workout ever devised. Scientifically proven advanced isometric exercises deliver a no-nonsense time-efficient workout that does everything you need to make your backside tight, firm, shapely and strong. No more time-wasting workouts where you twist, shake, and wiggle that might be fun but never deliver the results you want. Everyone has 60 seconds to spare, even on the busiest day, so, you are just 60 seconds a day from having a great ass. Required Equipment: 2 x Iso-Bows.

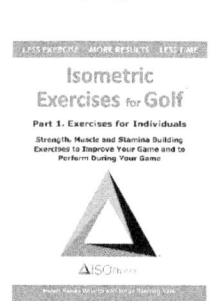

Isometric Exercises for Golf™ Part 1. Exercises for Individuals

This book has been approved by **TWiEA** – The World Isometric Exercise Association (www.TWiEA.com).

There is no such thing as a quick game of golf which means there is not always enough spare time to exercise in a gym as well. A series of advanced 7 to 10-second isometric exercises either while you play or practice is the answer. Perform just one isometric exercise at each hole and at the end of an 18-hole game you have completed a powerful total-body workout.

The average golf club is a perfect Improvised Isometric Exercise Device or IIED, so you are carrying your go-anywhere multi-gym everywhere you play. Part 1. is a resource guide of isometric exercises that can be performed by an individual. Note: The exercises in this book are either the same or similar to those in our books: Nordic Walking or Trekking Pole. The Isometric Exercises for Golf book 1 contains some special exercises designed to increase the strength and power of your golf swing.

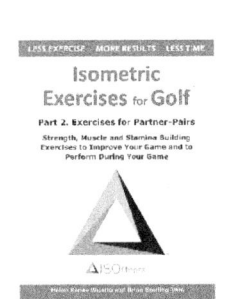

Isometric Exercises for Golf™ Part 2. Exercises for Partner-Pairs

This book has been approved by **TWiEA** – The World Isometric Exercise Association (www.TWiEA.com).

This is the companion to Book 1 and is focused on exercises that are best performed in partnered pairs, with a friend during a break, a game, or during practice sessions.

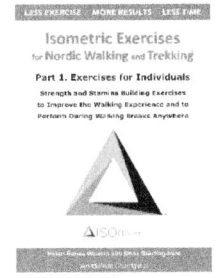

Isometric Exercises for Nordic Walking and Trekking™ - Part 1. Exercises for Individuals

This book has been approved by **TWiEA** – The World Isometric Exercise Association (www.TWiEA.com).

More Nordic Walkers and Trekkers than ever before perform proven gym-quality total-body isometric exercise routines during scheduled walk breaks in almost any location using their walking/trekking poles as an

IIED or Improvised Isometric Exercise Device. Book 1. is a resource guide of isometric exercises that can be performed as an individual, either outdoors or at home. Note: The exercises in this book are either the same or similar to those in our other books using a golf club. However, the Isometric Exercises for Golf book 1 contains some special exercises designed to increase the strength and power of your golf swing.

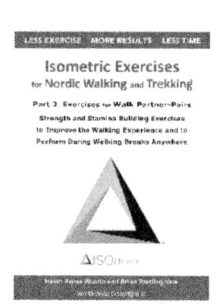

Isometric Exercises for Nordic Walking and Trekking™ - Part 2. Exercises for Walk Partner-Pairs

This book has been approved by **TWiEA** – The World Isometric Exercise Association (www.TWiEA.com).

This is the companion to Book 1 and is focused on exercises that are best performed as a partner-pair, with a friend during a walking break anywhere.

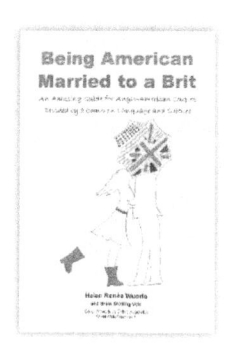

Being American Married to a Brit™ - An Amusing Guide for Anglo-American Couples Divided by a Common Language and Culture

When I first started dating my British man, I never gave a second thought about differences in language and culture. Why would I? After all, we Americans speak English, or do we…? As dating quickly turned into an engagement and then being married to my British gentleman, our common language and culture was a quirky, eye-opening, and highly amusing roller-coaster ride.

At times during the most basic everyday conversations, I would be listening to his words with glazed eyes, wondering what on earth he was saying. It was as if we were both speaking a different language. I decided to write this book and dedicate it to all transatlantic couples who will regularly find themselves completely divided and confused by their common language and culture.

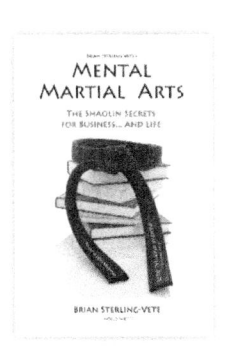

Mental Martial Arts™ - intellectual Life and Business Combat Skills
Brian Sterling-Vete's Mental Martial Arts is a system of intellectual life-combat skills using the tactics and principles of the physical martial arts. All interaction in life, business, and when communicating with others is an exchange of energy, power, and influence. Each party is always exerting maximum influence over the other to gain the outcome they prefer. The more powerful and persuasive will usually win unless the apparently weaker person is trained in Mental Martial Arts. You can learn how to verbally, intellectually, and emotionally guide, channel, and redirect the energy of others, even powerful people, and large organisations to more frequently achieve the outcomes that you desire in life and business. There is a section about how to handle a hostile news media in a crisis from experience gained over a decade with BBC TV News and a lifetime in martial arts to help you and your organisation stay Media Safe.

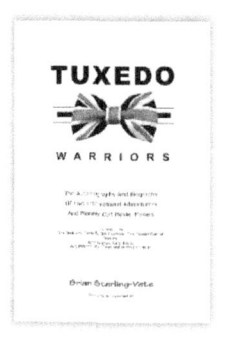

Tuxedo Warriors™

Tuxedo Warriors is the companion book to both The Tuxedo Warrior book and the movie. These books are the biography and autobiography of the iconic cult author, composer, and moviemaker Cliff Twemlow. The original book ended at the beginning of what has been called by many the Golden Age of Video Cinematography which Cliff inspired. Tuxedo Warriors continues the story from where his original book finishes, and it is the most complete biography of Cliff Twemlow ever written. It is also the autobiography of Brian Sterling-Vete who played a central role in this unique, entertaining, and true story of their adventures as guerrilla moviemakers.

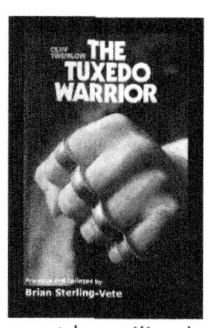

The Tuxedo Warrior™ by Cliff Twemlow – Prologue and epilogue by Brian Sterling-Vete.

There are many ways in which a Doorman can gain respect. Numerous methods were applied to the principle. In my profession, every available technique must be utilised, depending on the situation and circumstances. Would-be transgressors either move off the premises and quietly acknowledge your diplomatic approach. Or, the other alternative whereby physical persuasion must be exercised, which either quells their pugilistic desires or it triggers their aggressive instincts, turning the whole incident into a bloody and violent encounter. 'The Tuxedo Warrior,' pulls no punches in its brawling, savage, colourful, and entertaining exposure of society's nightlife activities.

The above is the original text from the rear cover of Cliff's book. Where his book finishes, my book *Tuxedo Warriors* begins to complete Cliff's colourful life story. I am honoured to be friends with Cliff's eldest son, Barry, and sincerely thank him for enabling this book and the others his father wrote to be re-published.

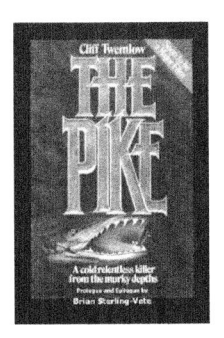

The Pike™ by Cliff Twemlow – Prologue and epilogue by Brian Sterling-Vete.

ITS FIRST VICTIMS - A screeching swan... A fisherman overboard... A drunken woman...

One by one, the mysterious killer in Lake Windermere claims its terrified victims. Tearing off limbs with its monstrous teeth, horribly mutilating bodies. Fear sweeps the peaceful holiday resort when experts identify the creature as a giant pike.... A hellish creature with the strength to rupture boats, and the anger to attack them. But for some, the terror becomes a bonanza—the traders who cater to the gathering crowds of ghouls on the shore. And they will do anything to stop divers from finding the creature. Meanwhile the ripples of bloodshed widen.... The Pike.

The above is the original text from the rear cover of Cliff's book which was to become a movie in the early 1980s starring Joan Collins.

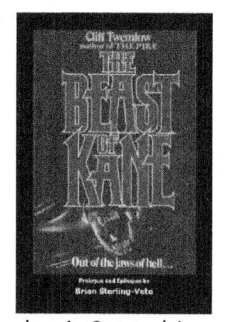

The Beast of Kane™ by Cliff Twemlow – Prologue and epilogue by Brian Sterling-Vete.

When the Gordon Family open their door to a stray Elkhound, they unwittingly welcome in the forces of evil. For, according to the local priest, the huge dog is Satan himself, fulfilling an ancient prophecy. But no one will believe this warning... Even when sheep – and wolves – are mysteriously slaughtered. Even when frenzied pets turn on their owners. Even when Emily Forrest is savagely eaten alive – the first of many human victims. As winter tightens its icy grip on the remote town of Kane, its unprotected people must face an unearthly terror.

The above is the original text from the rear cover of Cliff's book. This was the first of Cliff's books to be accepted by Hammer Film Studios to become a big-screen horror movie, along with Cliff's other book, The Pike.

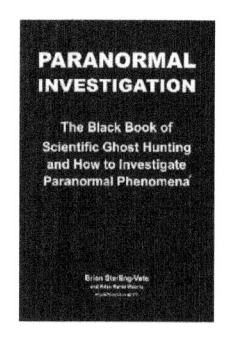

Paranormal Investigation - The Black Book of Scientific Ghost Hunting and How to Investigate Paranormal Phenomena™

This book is ideal for those who are new to paranormal investigation, and for more experienced investigators who want to learn more about how to apply a more scientific approach. It contains a special scientific critical path graphic page to work from when devising ghost-hunting experiments and to help train team members. There is a step-by-step guide to a complete paranormal investigation and vital information about how to protect yourself from malevolent paranormal entities that can attack you. It also contains ideas for potentially paranormally active and 'haunted' locations and several accounts of previously untold paranormal events including the remarkable Redwood Falls Minnesota UFO sighting.

The Haunting of Lilford Hall™ - The Birthplace of the United States as a Nation Haunted by the Man Behind The Pilgrim Fathers

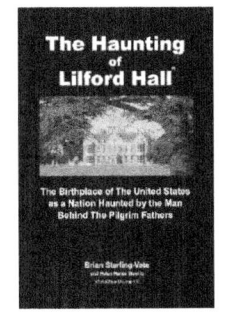

The Haunting of Lilford Hall is one of the most baffling cases ever recorded of paranormal activity experienced simultaneously by multiple people. Between 2012 and 2013, a team of 13 people produced a historical TV documentary about the life of Robert Browne, the man who was behind The Pilgrim Fathers sailing on The Mayflower to settle the first civilian colony on the American continent. Without Robert Browne, there may never have been the United States of America, at least not as we know it today. They experienced doors that refused to stay closed, they had debris thrown at them, and they had a door silently ripped away from the hinges and doorframe while they were in the next room. There were even several recorded multi-witness apparitions of a man fitting Robert Browne's recorded description. It is believed by many that the ghost of Robert Browne, the "Grandfather" of the United States as a nation, still haunts Lilford Hall.

- Robert Browne was the man who first separated the church from the state which is the underpinning of the United States.

- Robert Browne's words are written into the U.S. constitution.
- Robert Browne's direct descendent officially fired the first shot in the American war of independence.
- Robert Browne's beloved Lilford Hall estate was the home of President George Washington's mother home to President Quincy Adams' family.

www.MajorVision.com - www.TWiEA.com